Forgotten Disease

STUDIES OF THE WEATHERHEAD EAST
ASIAN INSTITUTE, COLUMBIA UNIVERSITY

The Studies of the Weatherhead East Asian Institute of Columbia University were inaugurated in 1962 to bring to a wider public the results of significant new research on modern and contemporary East Asia.

A complete list of titles is available online at weai.columbia.edu/ publications/studies-weai/.

Forgotten Disease

ILLNESSES TRANSFORMED IN
CHINESE MEDICINE

Hilary A. Smith

STANFORD UNIVERSITY PRESS

STANFORD, CALIFORNIA

Stanford University Press
Stanford, California

© 2017 by the Board of Trustees of the Leland Stanford Junior
University. All rights reserved.

Printed in the United States of America on acid-free, archival-
quality paper

Library of Congress Cataloging-in-Publication Data

Names: Smith, Hilary A., author.

Title: Forgotten disease : illnesses transformed in Chinese
    medicine / Hilary A. Smith.
Other titles: Studies of the Weatherhead East Asian Institute,
    Columbia University.
Description: Stanford, California : Stanford University Press,
    2017. | Series: Studies of the Weatherhead East Asian
    Institute, Columbia University | Includes bibliographical
    references and index.
Identifiers: LCCN 2017000968 | ISBN 9781503602090 (cloth :
    alk. paper) | ISBN 9781503603448 (pbk. : alk. paper) |
    ISBN 9781503603509 (epub)
Subjects: LCSH: Beri-beri—China—History. | Medicine—
    China—History. | Foot—Diseases—China—History. |
    Medical literature—China—History.
Classification: LCC RC627.B45 S45 2017 |
    DDC 610.951—dc23
LC record available at https://lccn.loc.gov/2017000968

Typeset by Thompson Type in 11/14 Adobe Garamond

Contents

Acknowledgments

It is a pleasure to thank some of those who made this book possible, even though these acknowledgments can't do justice to their generosity. My mentor Nathan Sivin has inspired my curiosity, modeled a scholarly life, and balanced critique with encouragement and humor. He has commented promptly and thoughtfully on draft after draft of my work. Everyone deserves such a mentor, but few are lucky enough to find one. David Barnes, Francesca Bray, and Victor Mair also provided insightful early feedback and crucial early-career support.

During a research stay in Beijing, I benefited from the expertise and guidance of Liao Yuqun, Zhang Daqing, Wang Shumin, and Sun Xiaochun, as well as the camaraderie and helpful suggestions of April Hongying Yin, Hu Yingchong, Zhou Libo, Ji Zhenghan, Sare Aricanli, and Priscilla Song. In Taiwan, Angela Leung and Chang Che-chia made my visit productive. My *shixiong* and *shijie*, Asaf Goldschmidt, Philip Cho, and Marta Hanson, led the way with encouragement, advice, and in Marta's case a binder full of relevant primary sources she had collected. Friends at Penn made drafts better and kept me going. I'm especially grateful to Emily Pawley, Babi Hammond, Eli Alberts, Paul Burnett, Josh Capitanio, Sungshin Kim, Cortney Chaffin, Rika Saito, Si Jia, Roger Turner, Erin McLeary, Sejal Patel, Tom Radice, Joy Rohde, Corinna Schlombs, Dominique Tobbell, Jeremy Vetter, and Ching-Jen Wang. At the Needham Research Institute, John Moffett helped me find sources and, along with Christopher Cullen, created a collegial and stimulating environment for hammering out ideas.

At Meredith and Dickinson Colleges and the University of Denver, colleagues and students have shown me why this stuff matters and helped craft it into a more readable form for a broader audience. I learned a lot from the questions they asked, the arguments that excited them, and the knowledge they'd developed through their own intellectual passions. Audra Wolfe of The Outside Reader handed me a paddle when the manuscript was bobbing somewhere between Research Island and the shores of Bookland. Since then, Wendy Jia-Chen Fu and Eric Karchmer have cheerfully read multiple drafts of the introduction and other parts of the book, and given me lots of new ideas. Bridie Andrews, Alex Bay, and two anonymous readers for Stanford University Press plowed through the entire manuscript (some of them twice!). They helped me avoid some embarrassing errors, rethink arguments, and articulate more clearly what I wanted to say. I owe them a great debt, and I alone am responsible for the shortcomings that remain.

It was Eugenia Lean who, after hearing about the project, suggested that it might fit well in the Weatherhead East Asian Institute series, and since then the supportive Ross Yelsey has helped steer it through its long journey. The editors and staff at Stanford University Press have guided this first-time author through the publishing process thoughtfully and professionally, including Kate Wahl, Olivia Bartz, and especially Jenny Gavacs, who saw potential in the manuscript and helped me figure out how to develop it. The Harvard-Yenching Institute and the China and Inner Asia Council of the Association for Asian Studies supported research trips to China and Taiwan. The University of Denver provided funds that paid for indexing and granted a one-quarter sabbatical that allowed me to complete the final revisions.

Two children and three new jobs followed the project's inception, so completing it has required heaps of moral and material support. Don and Jane Smith have given both unstintingly. And Babi Hammond keeps the whole ship afloat—even since learning how much bailing that involves. I couldn't ask for a better partner.

To all of the colleagues, companions, and institutions that have supported this endeavor, I am deeply grateful.

Forgotten Disease

Introduction

More than a few of the disease names we use today have been around for a long time, but what they mean now is different from what they meant hundreds of years ago. In English, for example, *cancer* was once a nonhealing sore caused by bodily humors congealing; *malaria* an intermittent fever caused by *mal aria*, bad air; and *influenza* severe seasonal fever, pain, and sniffles caused by the influence (hence the name) of unlucky stars. Now they are respectively an uncontrolled proliferation of cells, a fever caused by a mosquito-transmitted microbe, and a viral infection. Chinese speakers, too, use disease names that are many centuries old, such as sudden turmoil (*huo luan*) and flowers of heaven (*tian hua*), and the meanings of these names have likewise changed. Today sudden turmoil and flowers of heaven are equated with cholera and smallpox, but in the past they were systemic disruptions caused by invasive substances in the environment or by poison contracted in the womb.

This book examines the evolution of one Chinese disease concept, foot qi (*jiao qi*), from its origins in the fourth century to the present day. I use the word *evolution* in its neutral sense: not to indicate that the concept of foot qi has gotten better and better, more and more correct, but that it has changed over time to suit the intellectual, social, and epidemiological environment of the day. Contemporary biomedical scientists understand foot qi as the vitamin deficiency disease beriberi, but this view is no less peculiar and conditional than those that preceded and coexist with it, even if it has more cultural authority. To grasp the basic problem, let us examine three scenarios based on historical records of foot qi.

One: The Scholar's Scourge

Taizhou, southeast China, AD 1274. Che Ruoshui has been enjoying the life of a scholar, spending his days studying the classics, writing commentaries, and exchanging visits with other members of the local elite. When they gather they discuss philosophy, compose poems, and enjoy the finest food that the area has to offer, washed down by endless cups of rice wine. Che has attained notable career success, having studied with eminent teachers; the prefectural magistrate has appointed him to a post in the local academy and recommended him for other positions as well.

But in his mid-sixties Che finds himself crippled by a disease called foot qi. His feet swell and ache; he suffers piercing pain that makes it difficult to walk. Some doctors say his condition was caused by wind or wet qi common in this moist environment. He must have exposed himself to this qi by standing or sitting too long on the damp soil. Other doctors contend that by regularly drinking too much wine, he has damaged his spleen and stomach, impairing the normal circulation of his bodily energies and substances, leading to a stagnant circulation. Whatever the cause, foot qi is common in his social circle and is nothing to be ashamed of—in fact, it is a badge of his elite status. Che thus decides to title the philosophical meditations he is writing *Foot Qi Collectanea*, in ironic tribute to the disease that has immobilized him.[1]

Two: Dietary Disaster

Shinagawa, Japan, November 1884. The Japanese Imperial Navy's ship *Tsukuba* has returned from an eight-and-a-half-month voyage that took it to Hawaii, Russia, and Korea. During the voyage, fourteen men fell ill from a disease called foot qi (pronounced *kakke* in Japanese). They variously experienced swelling in the lower extremities, numbness, and heart palpitations. None died. This made *Tsukuba*'s brush with foot qi far more encouraging than that of her sister ship, *Ryūjō*, which had made the same voyage a year earlier. Nearly half of *Ryūjō*'s 376 men had contracted foot qi; twenty-five had died of it before the ship reached the halfway point in Hawaii. What saved the sailors on *Tsukuba* was a new regimen of rations that the Navy physician Takaki Kanehiro had put in place: more barley, less rice; more meat, less fish. The success of the new rations, combined with the observation that, unlike ordinary sailors, well-fed officers never get foot qi, convinces Takaki that the disease is caused by some sort of dietary imbalance or deficit.[2]

Three: A Formidable Fungus

Beijing today. A college student has unbearable itching between his toes, and a scaly rash has begun to spread along the balls of his feet—unmistakable signs of foot qi. Ugh! What a nuisance. He probably picked up the fungus in the communal showers or by borrowing his roommate's slippers. It's almost impossible to avoid the dreaded "Hong Kong foot" in modern life. That's why scenes like the one from the novel he's just been reading are so funny. One character uses the threat of foot qi to try to dissuade another from claiming the designer shoes that their mutual friend left behind:

> "Gao always had foot qi—a bad case—be careful you don't catch it when you wear those shoes."
> "No worries, no worries."
> "I once saw his feet were ulcerated, putting out pus."
> "How could it have been that bad? If it's really a problem I'll just wipe them with a little disinfectant."[3]

The Internet offers a whole arsenal of foot qi salves and ointments and sprays, so the student orders one he hopes will kill the fungus and take care of the problem. He vows to keep his feet clean and dry and never to borrow slippers again.

* * *

Foot qi, a two-character compound in the Chinese script that speakers of Chinese, Korean, and Japanese have all shared, has appeared in East Asian texts since at least the fourth century AD. But, as these three scenarios show, the term has meant very different things in different periods and places. In some contexts, foot qi was a goutlike affliction of the well-to-do, painful but not generally fatal; in others, foot qi was beriberi, which disproportionately struck the lower classes, killed swiftly, and was caused by a nutritional deficiency. In mainland China today, foot qi is athlete's foot, the itchy scourge of public showers. It afflicts many but kills no one.

How can we reconcile these vignettes? They use the same name for what, from a modern biomedical perspective, are clearly different conditions. The most common approach is to privilege the middle one over the other two, to say that what afflicted Japanese sailors in the nineteenth century was *true* foot qi, whereas the sufferers in the other two scenarios really had something else, even if the victims or their doctors didn't recognize it.[4] Meanings of foot qi that predated microbiology are deemed too unscientific, and the current athlete's foot meaning too colloquial, to accept as legitimate readings. So foot qi is *really*, historians and scientists tell us, beriberi.

The problem is that privileging a nineteenth-century translation like this distorts our understanding of the past. It places undue emphasis on discoveries made by Western and Western-trained physicians in the nineteenth century, ignoring the extensive body of premodern Chinese medical literature. It prioritizes the kinds of suffering characteristic of the dawn of the modern age and recognizes the suffering of past invalids only to the extent that it resembles that outmoded model. It closes off alternative readings of ancient medical texts, limiting the applications of the knowledge those texts contain. And it ignores scholarship in the history of medicine showing how social and cultural environments shape disease concepts.

If such historical myopia were unique to foot qi, one could dismiss it as an oddity. But it is not. Many other ancient diseases, such as flowers of heaven (*tian hua*), sudden turmoil (*huo luan*), plum poison (*mei du*), and numbing wind (*ma feng*), are similarily distorted by the translations they acquired in the modern period: respectively and unambiguously, smallpox, cholera, syphilis, and leprosy. The consequences appear in historical depictions both popular and scholarly: in *Red Cliff* (*Chi Bi*), a movie based on historical events of the third century BC, soldiers in camp are afflicted by a disease called cold damage (*shang han*), which the English subtitles translate "typhoid."[5] The translation, based on an association between *shang han* and typhoid developed in the nineteenth century and reinforced, as Sean Hsianglin Lei has shown, in the 1930s, confers unwarranted precision on the ancient epidemic.[6] It may be unreasonable to expect to see historical best practices in a blockbuster film, but specialized historical sources elide modern and ancient illnesses in the same way. A recent scholarly translation of the Chinese medical classic *The Yellow Emperor's Inner Canon*, produced by experienced specialists in the field of Chinese medical history, straightforwardly translates the ancient term *nüe* as "malaria," even though, as the translators themselves concede, *nüe* at this time was probably used for "all types of intermittent fevers."[7] By contrast, the same scholars allow terms that did not acquire a modern translation in the late nineteenth or early twentieth century—such as *jie*, which also indicated an intermittent fever—to remain untranslated. Thus the translated text implies that historians understand what the *Inner Canon*'s *nüe* was better than we understand what its *jie* was.[8] We don't.

This book argues that we need a more satisfactory way to approach premodern Chinese diseases. It offers a history of one such disease, the one called foot qi, to provide an example of what a better approach might look like. Foot qi epitomizes the problem of presentist translation. It features in thousands of pre–twentieth-century medical books, and the diversity of symptoms associated with it makes it impossible to identify foot qi with a single modern disease. Chinese and Japanese sources written before the nineteenth century describe it as a protean ailment that mostly plagued the rich and sedentary. In some cases the feet and lower legs swelled up, some were accompanied by chills and fever, and some featured shortness of breath. Some foot qi sufferers are described as feeling "a creeping sensation like insects crawling around" or "a thing like fingers . . . which travels upward and attacks the heart."[9] They might be particularly sensitive to cold, to light, or to the smell of food; they might have twitching in the lower legs or across the entire body. Hot flashes and headaches plagued some foot qi patients, whereas some experienced stomach pain and throbbing in the chest. Sources mention both dementia and diarrhea as diagnostic signs. An eighteenth-century text illustrates "foot qi sores" on the calves, filled with yellow fluid, as a signature (see Figure 4 in Chapter Seven). And this is hardly a comprehensive list of signs.

One might expect such variety in the sources to stymie attempts to identify foot qi with a single modern disease. Without the blood and urine tests available today to measure vitamin levels in the body, it is impossible to confidently say that the diverse symptoms associated with foot qi in the premodern literature were clinical beriberi. Some of the described symptoms, to be sure, match those of modern beriberi: lower leg swelling and weakening, for example, or heart palpitations and dementia in advanced cases. Others do not, including chills and fever, sores, or the crawling-insect sensations. And even those symptoms that are a good match are too diffuse and general to rule out other possibilities. As the contemporary historian Liao Yuqun has suggested, heart disease, syphilis, and heavy metal poisoning fit equally well and, in some instances, better.[10] Gout, too, corresponds well to descriptions of foot qi in certain periods, as Chapter Five shows.

Despite this pile of credible alternatives, however, it is the vitamin deficiency disorder beriberi that stands aloft as the officially sanctioned translation of foot qi, past and present, as a look at any Chinese dictionary will attest. Occasionally athlete's foot rates a secondary mention as an "informal" meaning of the term, but beriberi is consistently the first and approved meaning. Even the venerable *Great Dictionary of Chinese* (*Han yu da ci dian*), which traces the historical etymology of classical Chinese words as the *Oxford English Dictionary* does for English ones, defines foot qi as "A disease caused by a deficiency of vitamin B1," although the third-century usage example that follows this definition does not indicate such a deficiency. The standard translation also affects the way librarians classify old books: one Library of Congress subject heading for the eleventh-century *Comprehensive Essentials for the Treatment of Foot Qi* is "Beri-beri—treatment—early works to 1800."

This book explores the history of foot qi in seven chronologically ordered chapters. Chapter One examines the context in which Chinese observers first began to write about foot qi in the fourth century CE. At a time when conflict was driving large numbers of Chinese aristocrats from their homes on the north China plain southward to the Yangzi River area, foot qi seemed to be a particular problem of northern emigrants facing southern miasmas. Their bodies were not prepared to confront the foreign environment of their new home. Chapter Two shows how seventh-century rival healers and patients themselves disagreed about foot qi's causes, symptoms, and appropriate treatment, reflecting the unregulated and competitive medical occupation characteristic of imperial China. Chapter Three explains how, in the tenth century, a government unusually active in promoting public health standardized and simplified foot qi in ways that would eventually carry over into modern categories of beriberi. Chapter Four investigates how a thirteenth-century physician fascinated by digestion created a new form of foot qi related to bad diet, and Chapter Five analyzes the social and economic circumstances that turned that new dietary disorder into the most prominent form of the disease in late imperial China. In Chapter Six you will find the story of beriberi's rise in Asia and how foot qi and the vitamin deficiency disorder came to be treated as synonyms in nineteenth-century Japan. Finally, Chapter Seven shows how the modernizing elite in early twentieth-century China accepted the Japanese reinterpretation of foot qi as beriberi and how most Chinese people, who had little experience of beriberi, rejected that definition in favor of one more personally relevant: athlete's foot.

Even in the age of biomedicine, concepts of foot qi remain complex. In Japan, it is understood as beriberi; in Taiwan, usually as beriberi but sometimes as athlete's foot; and in mainland China, sometimes as beriberi, usually as athlete's foot, and occasionally a goutlike pain disorder. These differences are rooted in the very different paths of transformation that each East Asian nation followed in the early twentieth century, and they belie the impression that the biomedical translation of a classical East Asian disease concept is bound to be universal.

Framing Disease: Extending and Defending the Approach

When it comes to the history of disease, ideas from the late nineteenth and early twentieth centuries have particular inertia. That is the period when the cornerstone of modern scientific medicine—also called biomedicine—was laid. Concepts developed at that time are part of the edifice of biomedicine: evolution, germ theory, vitamins and nutritional deficiency disorders, genes. Concepts that predate it are not: humors, miasma, demonic possession, and divine curses. This oversimplifies what was in fact a complex and gradual transition, of course, but it accurately describes the seminal importance of the late nineteenth century in contemporary understandings of medical history.

According to the medical historian Charles Rosenberg, the nineteenth century fostered a revolution in the way Western physicians and patients understood illness. Just as profound as the contemporaneous Darwinian revolution that encouraged people to think about all living things as related and derived from a common source, what Rosenberg calls the "specificity revolution" fostered the idea that disease is an entity in itself, separable from sick people. A disease, in this *ontological* way of thinking, had a single specific cause, an identifiable physical mechanism, and a predictable clinical course, regardless of the idiosyncrasies of the person or environment in which it appeared.[11] Although some physicians, notably Thomas Sydenham, had espoused a similar idea centuries earlier, for the most part Western doctors before the nineteenth century thought of disease *physiologically*, holding that the peculiarities of a patient and her milieu made her condition unique.[12] In this older way of thinking, a case of syphilis might turn into leprosy—conceived of not as different diseases but as the continuation of a single illness experience—and the same disease might well have different causes.[13] After the specificity revolution, such things were no longer possible.

Today, it has become very difficult to escape the ontological way of thinking. New diagnostic technologies, the complexity of hospital care, and the bureaucratic regimes associated with hospitals, insurance companies, and public health departments have conspired to make a standard diagnosis indispensable. To be ill today is to submit to what Rosenberg calls the "tyranny of diagnosis"—to depend on and be defined by a diagnosis. Hence, most people think of disease as a thing in itself, something that has an existence and a coherent identity of its own; sick people are its victims. We talk in all sincerity about fighting wars against AIDS, malaria, or even cancer, as if they were enemies ranged on a battlefield somewhere outside of our bodies. And because, by dint of imperialism and inspiration, what in the nineteenth century was Western medicine has spread to other parts of the world and become global biomedicine, the ontological perspective reigns in China today as well.[14] It is difficult to see around a concept so deeply embedded in contemporary thought.

Nevertheless, in the 1990s historians began to find their way past the ontological perspective. Inspired by social constructionists who argued that what most people consider natural categories are actually defined by human minds and reflect their experiences and culture, students of the past approached diseases as both natural phenomena and cultural concepts. Diagnosis was thus a process of "framing" disease, making it a legible social entity; investigating the framing process could reveal a great deal about the society in which sick people lived and died.[15] This approach undercut the presumed naturalness of contemporary diagnoses such as end-stage renal disease and coronary heart disease, showing the messy social process by which they'd been transformed from older, but no more arbitrary, identities.[16] It enabled the historian Jeremy Greene to show how therapeutic tools developed over the past few decades have changed the American understanding of what constitutes disease; having drugs that effectively lower blood cholesterol, for example, has made asymptomatic high cholesterol itself a pathological condition to be treated, which it never could have been before.[17] Importantly, this approach also persuaded historians to resist applying contemporary diagnoses to historical illnesses. Because today's diagnoses are as influenced by today's prejudices and preconceptions as previous diagnoses had been by those of the past, imposing our categories on our predecessors' experiences is simple presentism. As Andrew Cunningham has put it, "You die of what your doctor says you die of," even if that is something as unfamiliar to later minds as "rising of the lights" is to us today. No one, looking back, can gainsay the diagnoses of the past.[18]

The present book both extends and defends the "framing" approach to disease. It extends the approach to Chinese disease concepts, which have not undergone the kind of rigorous historical deconstruction that biomedical disease concepts have. In part this is because historians of Western medicine have evinced little interest in Chinese medicine. In part it is because many present-day proponents of Chinese medicine are no keener to see their narrative of an unchanging tradition challenged than biomedical physicians have been to see their narrative of unceasing progress undermined. Where *longue-durée* narratives about China take disease as a central focus, they generally use a biomedical disease concept as the starting point and definition of what they're investigating, purporting to offer a history of leprosy or smallpox, for example, from ancient times to the present.[19] Other histories of disease in China simply eschew the longitudinal approach, instead beginning with the nineteenth century when we can be reasonably sure that what the sources label "sudden turmoil" really *was* what a physician today would recognize as cholera, and that the epidemics the historian identifies as bubonic plague really were the bacillus-caused disease we call bubonic plague today.[20] I prefer to follow the example of historians who resist imposing modern categories, generally Western derived, on premodern Chinese forms of knowledge. Benjamin Elman, for instance, judges premodern Chinese science according to its practitioners' own objectives and not by how closely it approximated what Western scientists were doing at the same time.[21] Similarly, Marta Hanson explores changing ideas about *wen bing*, warm diseases, without reducing them to the Chinese equivalent of a biomedical disease category.[22] This book likewise seeks to present traditional Chinese concepts of disease and healing on their own terms.

In addition to expanding the purview of cultural histories of disease, it now seems necessary to defend them. Today, historians continue to reinforce the tyranny of diagnosis. Although no historian of medicine would now suggest that modern diagnoses represent unmediated biological reality, many other scholars uncritically apply the ontological perspective. The most widely read histories of disease stick so confidently to that perspective, in fact, that they present diseases as actors—not merely beings that can attack people but beings that can change the course of history. Following in the footsteps of William McNeill and Alfred Crosby, recent histories have investigated how disease inhibited or facilitated human colonization of particular environments, how and when disease spread from one geographical region to another, and especially how disease influenced the outcome of conflict among different peoples.[23] In such histories, the identities of the diseases in question are invariably modern biomedical identities and almost invariably acute infectious diseases whose causative microorganism is known: plague, yellow fever, influenza, smallpox.

The best specimens of this sort of scholarship are fascinating and tell us important things about evolution and epidemiology. They synthesize scientific, archaeological, and historical evidence impressively. By showing how much biotas matter, they also invalidate arguments that the distribution of power and wealth in the modern world—disproportionately concentrated in what Crosby calls the "neo-Europes," where people of European descent predominate—reflects the cultural and intellectual superiority of the rich and powerful. In other words, these histories make useful contributions to understanding.

They do not tell us much of interest about people, however. Global histories of disease tend to discount or ignore altogether the way in which people in the past understood and managed their own suffering, in the process foreclosing other ways in which we, today, might understand our own.[24] The irony is that the kinds of illnesses that contemporary readers are most liable to experience themselves are not the acute infectious diseases that these histories focus on but chronic noncommunicable disorders that are less well understood.

When it comes to the kinds of ills that kill most of us today, treating disease history as if it were military history in which humans combat disease (or sometimes ally themselves with disease against other humans) encourages simplistic and unproductive thinking. If cancer is a proliferation of our own rogue cells, is a war against it a war against ourselves?

Foot qi is just the sort of chronic noncommunicable ailment that most disease history has ignored. Most of the historical records on foot qi—the late nineteenth-century epidemics aside—do not present it as the sort of disease that felled large numbers of people all at once, decimating armies or cities. Foot qi was experienced, instead, as episodes of pain and weakness that might afflict an individual intermittently over the course of years or even a lifetime. Someone who was unlucky enough to be diagnosed or treated improperly might be killed by either the disorder or the treatment. But for most, foot qi was just a chronic nuisance. One cannot cast such disorders in starring roles in world-changing conflict or the collapse of civilizations. Still, they do help us understand how some people made sense of and managed pedestrian kinds of suffering that may be more universal.

If "the disease that changed world history" narratives represent the persistence of the ontological perspective, the biographies-of-disease genre is its apotheosis. "Biographies" of cancer, cholera, malaria, diabetes, AIDS, and many other diseases have appeared in bookstores and libraries over the past few years. Some are more sophisticated than others in their awareness of how social and cultural context have shaped contemporary medical concepts. But even the most nuanced help naturalize the ontological view; the very idea of a disease biography implies that the disease at its center is real and has an independent existence and a life story one can trace.[25] As the historian of medicine Roger Cooter points out, this sort of exercise

> is foremost an engagement with the present, not the past. The illusion is that the history of a disease is being related, whereas in reality, the present understanding of the disease is being confirmed. It is our biological knowledge of disease that is in the driving seat, not the pursuit of any historical understanding.[26]

Displacing contemporary knowledge of disease from the driver's seat means paying attention to ideas important to the people who experienced and treated the illnesses of the past. In the case of foot qi, this includes ideas about wind poison, inherently toxic locales, and spleen depletion that would be seen as quaint misapprehensions if the ultimate destination of this history were beriberi. But this book does not seek to explain the history of beriberi in China; instead, it shows how and why Chinese concepts of a single disease changed over time. It advocates, in short, treating disease not as an actor but as what it is: an experience whose meaning and parameters people define—and contest.

Diversity and Change in Chinese Medical History

Recent histories of Chinese medicine have conveyed a sense of its diversity, how ideas and practices that fall under its rubric vary in different cultural contexts, across different socioeconomic levels, and in different periods.[27] Chinese medicine in the contemporary United States differs from Chinese medicine in contemporary China; the medicine practiced by an elite amateur in late imperial China differed from the medicine practiced by a less-educated hereditary herbalist; and Chinese doctors of the second century BC both thought and practiced differently from Chinese doctors of the eighteenth century. None of this should surprise a student of history, attuned to change over time as well as difference across and within cultures. But Chinese medicine is particularly vulnerable to essentialization, to being presented as ancient, unified, and unchanging. This is because Chinese medicine, unlike classical Western medicine, boasts a significant community of modern proponents and practitioners. A historian who examines premodern Western perspectives on illness—how humoral imbalance and exposure to miasma might precipitate malaria, for example—is dealing with a set of ideas that almost no one now espouses.[28] By contrast, there are multitudes of healers in China and around the world who claim to apply and transmit premodern Chinese ideas.

The existence of such a robust community is, on the one hand, a great boon to the historian; it fuels the editing, annotation, and republication of numerous classical medical sources useful to her research and widens the audience for her own scholarship. Interacting with practitioners also helps her bear in mind the real challenges that healers in any age face as they attempt to grapple with people and illnesses in all their complexity. But the narratives about Chinese medicine's history that practitioners propagate can be misleading. Because modern Chinese medicine has developed in the shadow of biomedicine, in places struggling to avoid being stamped out, its advocates have sometimes adopted defensive postures that cause them to present premodern Chinese medical knowledge as unchanged since antiquity and diametrically different from Western medicine, two perspectives that careful historical study cannot support.

To defend Chinese medicine in societies where faith in biomedicine is strong, its proponents have settled on a kind of division of labor, emphasizing differences in worldview, diagnosis, and treatment. Chinese medicine, they say, focuses on process and function, whereas biomedicine focuses on structure and composition; thus, the study of anatomy, central to biomedicine, is peripheral to Chinese medicine.[29] Chinese medicine is holistic and takes into account the entire body as well as the whole person in her environment; Western medicine is reductionistic and concerned with ever-smaller units—organs, tissues, cells, molecules.[30] Chinese medicine is good for chronic diseases whereas biomedicine is good for acute infectious diseases.[31] Chinese medicine views the body as an ecosystem to be maintained in dynamic equilibrium, unlike Western medicine, which views it as a battleground on which we must kill invading pathogens.[32] Because each is strong where the other is weak, there is room for both, even a *necessity* for both, in modern societies where health-care resources are scarce.

Although this contrastive approach has been fairly successful as a survival strategy—in China, Chinese medicine is widespread and state supported alongside biomedicine, and it is increasingly recognized and practiced in other parts of the world too[33]—it distorts our impression of both Chinese and Western medicine before the twentieth century, as historians are demonstrating. Consider the chronic-versus-acute distinction. In the early twentieth century, practitioners of Chinese medicine did not think of their art as especially applicable to chronic diseases; in fact, many of the Republican-era doctors the anthropologist Eric Karchmer has interviewed reported that they and their teachers built their reputations on success at treating acute diseases. They report, moreover, that they were more likely to see patients with acute problems than with chronic conditions; most people didn't call in a doctor for symptoms that they thought they could endure.[34] And Western medicine before sulfa drugs and antibiotics, it must be added, was unimpressive when it came to treating acute infectious diseases. Likewise, as regards structure-versus-function, the historian Yi-Li Wu has shown that some prominent nineteenth-century Chinese physicians, contrary to the common understanding today, took a keen interest in anatomy, while some Western physicians of the same period questioned the importance of anatomical knowledge to medical practice.[35] Like the chronic-versus-acute distinction, this one sharpened later, as the two forms of medicine developed side by side. Similarly, Shigehisa Kuriyama has shown in early Chinese medical texts "a science ruled as much by martial images of siege and invasion as by the holistic ideals of balance and harmony," contrary to today's perception that metaphors of sickness-as-war are foreign to this tradition.[36]

Modern changes in Chinese medicine have similarly distorted premodern concepts of Chinese disease. Here is how one of the most influential Western-language introductions to Chinese medicine, Ted Kaptchuk's *The Web That Has No Weaver*, describes the way a practitioner of Chinese medicine views illness, in contrast to the way a biomedical physician does. The practitioner of Chinese medicine

> directs his or her attention to the complete physiological and psychological individual. All relevant information, including the symptoms as well as the patient's other general characteristics, is gathered and woven together until it forms what Chinese medicine calls a "pattern of disharmony." This pattern of disharmony describes a situation of "imbalance" in a patient's body. Oriental diagnostic technique does

not turn up a specific disease entity or a precise cause, but renders an almost poetic, yet workable, description of the whole person.[37]

Biomedical physicians care about diseases; Chinese medicine practitioners care about "patterns of disharmony." Kaptchuk goes on to describe a situation in which six patients diagnosed by biomedical doctors as having peptic ulcer disease are diagnosed with six different patterns of disharmony by six different Chinese medicine doctors—highlighting, he says, the Chinese medicine doctors' attention to the uniqueness of each person.

But classical Chinese medical texts do not only discuss patterns of disharmony. They are full of *bing* too, and in many cases "disease" seems precisely the right way to translate this term: often, the authors present a *bing* as caused by an invasive substance, manifesting a consistent set of symptoms and having a predictable clinical course. In places, classical Chinese texts express ontological views of illness; in other places, they express more physiological views—just as the Western medical tradition included both Sydenham's specific diseases and Rudolf Virchow's contention that "Disease is nothing but life under altered conditions."[38] It can be difficult, however, to see disease-as-entity in the Chinese sources when contemporary practitioners insist that such a notion is alien to the tradition.

What Kaptchuk articulates is a distinction that, as Volker Scheid has shown, was crafted in the 1950s. Before the twentieth century, "disease," "pattern" and "symptom" coexisted in classical Chinese medicine, and no rigorous attempt was made to differentiate them from one another; in Scheid's words, "No unequivocal or dominant nosological system ever emerged during the classical era."[39] The 1930s saw attempts by both the Nationalist government and reformers within Chinese medicine to accept Western disease concepts as valid and tie Chinese disease concepts to them.[40] These efforts failed to gain traction among practitioners of Chinese medicine, who reasonably saw such equivalences as a kind of capitulation, according Western medicine the authority to define what disease really was. In the 1950s, as Chinese medicine spasmodically made its way to a secure place in the new People's Republic of China, political and professional agendas converged to turn "determining treatments [through] pattern differentiation" (*bian zheng lun zhi*) into the signature approach of traditional medicine. The idea that Chinese medicine *differentiated patterns* (*bian zheng*) rather than diagnosing diseases appealed to practitioners worried about whether the new government would allow Chinese medicine to persist (health policy, like so much else in the early PRC, was subject to sudden and unpredictable change).[41] It appealed in part because it fit well with Communist ideology; the term was a homophone with "dialectical materialism" (also *bian zheng*) and implied that Chinese medicine doctors' diagnostic process involved analyzing and synthesizing opposites, in good Hegelian fashion. It also appealed because it had become clear by the 1930s that traditional Chinese disease concepts could not compete with Western ones in a world epidemiologically dominated by infectious disease and intellectually dominated by the laboratory.[42] Classical theories of causation—wind, damp, excessive anger—sounded primitive compared to the claims of microbiology, backed by photographs of bacteria as seen through high-powered microscopes. And although some scientists praised ancient Chinese physicians for creating vitamin-rich prescriptions centuries before anyone knew about vitamins, by the time synthetic vitamins were available such old prescriptions were of mainly antiquarian interest.[43] With the advent of antibiotics it became even clearer that focusing on how classical doctors had understood and treated *diseases* would not keep Chinese medicine alive as a vibrant, viable healing art. Modern Western medicine had infectious disease well in hand (or so it seemed, mid-century). Classical *bing* that had been identified with particular microbes and vitamin deficiencies in the previous decades, therefore, were marginalized in modern Chinese medicine, ceded to Western medicine in its "golden age."[44] Foot qi gradually disappeared from textbooks used at Traditional Chinese Medicine (TCM) colleges in the People's Republic of China.[45] Today TCM physicians are required to use biomedical categories to report diagnoses on workers' documentation.

This book contributes to the blurring of the distinctions between Chinese and Western medicine that have sharpened, since the late nineteenth century, until they have come to look like absolute qualities of contrasting modes of healing. It seeks to highlight the diversity in the Chinese medical canon. Chinese medicine practitioners before the modern period *did* sometimes think about diseases ontologically, as consistently recognizable in different people and caused by invasive pathogens. They saw patterns of disharmony in sick bodies, yes, but they also saw diseases, and one of the ones they saw was foot qi. When Western-trained doctors came along suggesting that foot qi was a vitamin deficiency disorder, the contrast was not between people who saw disease and people who saw patterns of disharmony. It was between people who had different understandings of what caused a condition and how to treat it.

By calling attention to an aspect of the tradition that has been neglected or excluded as Chinese medicine has modernized, the story of foot qi contributes to the more complex picture of the modern relationship between Chinese and Western medicine that has recently begun to emerge. Bridie Andrews, Sean Hsiang-lin Lei, Volker Scheid, and others have replaced an old impression of medicine in modern China as an encounter between a Chinese tradition unchanged since ancient times and an inquisitive, dynamic Western science.[46] In its place, they have shown us an early twentieth-century environment in which the meanings of "Chinese" and "Western" medicine were themselves inchoate. These broad rubrics obscure variety—"Western" medicine, for example, could mean French medicine, Anglo-American medicine, German medicine, and Japanese medicine, each distinctive[47]—and rapid change. Both forms of healing were evolving in tandem and would continue to do so over the course of the twentieth century.[48] Lei uses the metaphor of speciation to capture this dynamic: the early twentieth century was not a time when a traditional medicine somehow survived an onslaught by modern medicine but rather a time in which a new species, Chinese medicine, began to evolve in the peculiar political, intellectual, and social environment of Republican China (and, perhaps, another new species in the form of Chinese Western medicine—but no one has yet studied how this same peculiar environment shaped local biomedicine).[49] Republican China did not see the clash of a modern medicine with a traditional one; it saw the sprouts of two new modern forms of healing emerging side by side.

The story of foot qi reflects this diversity and change: nineteenth- and twentieth-century discussions of foot qi were not examples of a fully formed Western idea about vitamin deficiency butting up against a longstanding Chinese idea about wind poison or dietary surfeit. Classical Chinese doctors had multiple ideas about foot qi, and Western-style doctors were actively fumbling their way toward the concepts of vitamins and supplementation. Concepts were still in formation on all sides, and some ideas from premodern foot qi literature (such as the notion that there were wet, dry, and fulminant forms) found their way into beriberi literature just as ideas about beriberi entered that of foot qi. Moreover, diversity has persisted: some people today understand foot qi as a vitamin deficiency disorder, others understand it as a foot fungus, and still others understand it as a foot fungus that can be *cured* with vitamin supplements—a curious hybridization. What's more, people in other parts of East Asia understand the term differently from people in mainland China, divergences that, as Chapter Seven shows, reflect the different modern trajectories of Japan, Taiwan, Korea, and mainland China. In sum, the story of foot qi further complicates the popular notion of a monolithic and unchanging Chinese medicine that contrasts consistently with Western medicine.

Disease and Imperialism

The book also contributes to destabilizing old narratives about the spread of Western power and its effect on global health. The way scholars think about disease outside of Europe and America—and the European and American role in shaping the global disease burden—has changed a great deal. In the eighteenth and nineteenth centuries, Europeans expanding their influence and possessions overseas encountered diseases that they were either unfamiliar with or that were much deadlier and more widespread in the colonies than they were at home in Europe: smallpox, malaria, yellow fever, sleeping sickness, kala-azar, and the like. This led many nineteenth-century Western observers to suppose that the non-European world was by nature a sick one and that the diseases inherent there impeded Western colonization.[50]

Western settlers nonetheless believed they could heal this sick world by bringing more advanced medicine and technology, more civilized lifestyles, and truer religious beliefs than those present before their arrival. With their aid, no longer would Africa and Asia be ravaged by illnesses that Europeans saw as the result of ignorance and immorality. As Rudyard Kipling declared, an important part of the "white man's burden" was to "bid the sickness cease."[51]

The paternalism that Kipling and other nineteenth-century writers expressed faded as empires receded. By the 1970s and 1980s, historians were exploring how European expansion had introduced disease to native populations, in addition to sometimes relieving it. McNeill and Crosby examined how microbes that European settlers transported across the Atlantic helped depopulate the Americas, showing that infectious disease had not been an impediment to European expansion in every case.[52] At the end of the century this understanding had spread to the popular imagination; widely read books such as Jared Diamond's *Guns, Germs and Steel* argued that the biological arsenal Europeans unwittingly carried helped them conquer the globe.[53] Still, this newer analysis centered on infectious diseases such as smallpox and typhus and did not dislodge the belief that other ailments—parasitic and vector-borne diseases such as kala-azar and malaria and nutritional deficiencies like beriberi—had indeed blighted most of Africa and Asia long before European arrival.

More recently, however, historians have begun to argue that it was not just by introducing microbes to populations unaccustomed to them that European imperialists changed the disease burden in Asia, Africa, and the Americas. The social and economic changes that Westerners wrought there mattered equally. David S. Jones has argued that Indians died of smallpox in large numbers not because they were "virgin soil" for the virus, as older histories would have it, but because Europeans dispossessed them of their land and disrupted their patterns of obtaining food. This left the Indians malnourished and more vulnerable to infectious disease. In addition, indiscriminate slaughter had rendered small communities unable to properly care for the sick as they had in the past.[54] Similarly, Christian McMillen has questioned the old (and recently revived) idea that Indians were more genetically susceptible to tuberculosis than whites in the early twentieth century, suggesting that the squalor and deprivation of reservation life had more to do with their high rates of death from the disease.[55] This line of inquiry has led scholars to reexamine the effects of Western imperialism on other kinds of diseases, those previously assumed to have been features of Asian and African life from time immemorial. As it turns out, mosquito-borne infections such as malaria also owed much to colonial activity. Clearing and irrigating land for agriculture created new pools of stagnant water in which mosquitoes could breed; the poor living conditions of plantation workers exposed them to mosquitoes and degraded their immune defenses; and the mass migrations of people—some malaria infected—that the Western presence provoked spread the parasite to new areas. Starting in the nineteenth century, as Randall Packard has shown, malaria thus spread from a local problem found in many pockets of the world to become endemic to the tropics.[56] The case of malaria in the Panama Canal Zone is a particularly illuminating example of how complex the relationship between Western imperialism and global disease was. It is well known that the American army physician William Gorgas managed to curb devastating epidemics of these diseases in the Zone in 1904 through a concerted mosquito eradication campaign. Less frequently observed is how the canal project itself had fueled the epidemics, as poorly nourished laborers slept outdoors next to the water-logged, mosquito-breeding ditches that they themselves were digging![57] As for parasitic diseases such as kala-azar, bilharzia, and sleeping sickness, the medical historian Roy Porter concluded that they

> were not features waiting to be discovered, like the source of the Nile; they had often been aggravated or even created by imperialism. Bringing war, the flight of people, clearings, settlements, encampments, roads and railways and other ecological disruptions, and the reduction of native populations to wage-labour or to marginal lands, colonization spread disease.[58]

Historians have not yet subjected the relationship between nutritional deficiency disorders and nineteenth-century imperialism to this kind of analysis. Newer histories of nutritional deficiency disorders and vitamins still present the former as a timeless scourge finally resolved by the latter. "The empire building and colonization activities of Western Europe's powerful nations during the sixteenth to the nineteenth centuries," writes the author of a recent history of vitamin A, "inevitably, if slowly, awakened the industrialized West to health conditions in impoverished parts of Asia and Africa." This suggests that what was new in the age of imperialism was Western *awareness* of health conditions that had been a perennial feature of poor agricultural societies.[59] The title of a book on beriberi sums up this triumphant approach well: *Beriberi, White Rice, and Vitamin B: A Disease, a Cause, and a Cure.*[60] There are hints in these histories that epidemic-scale nutritional deficiency diseases were new in the nineteenth and early twentieth centuries, but such glimpses tend to be incidental and quickly passed over.[61]

This history of foot qi suggests that the beriberi outbreaks of the nineteenth century were, in fact, a new phenomenon that reflected the rise of imperialism and industrialization just as surely as did the large-scale epidemics of smallpox, typhus, tuberculosis, and malaria in the same period. Reframing beriberi as but one change in foot qi's long story highlights the novelty of those nineteenth-century conditions. In this way, the study contributes to the more complex and more accurate understanding that is currently forming of how the modern distribution of power helped shape the global disease burden and how Western medicine reinforced imperial hierarchies at the same time that it relieved some illnesses.[62]

* * *

In short, this book aims to convince you that it is time to reread the histories of non-Western disease names translated into modern medical terms in the late nineteenth and early twentieth centuries, understanding that period as but one among a number of transformative episodes in the long histories of these concepts. Doing so will illuminate what was lost and gained as Chinese and Western medicine coevolved in the late nineteenth and early twentieth centuries. It will challenge the assumption that Western medical knowledge solved long-standing, intractable health problems in East Asia. Most important, it will help us escape the tyranny of diagnosis by highlighting how past perceptions of the body, health, and illness differed from those of today. Such an effort may even enable us to imagine suffering differently in the present, expanding our current repertoire of ways to think about human experience.

CHAPTER ONE

Foot Qi in Early Chinese Medicine

The year is AD 313. An official of the Jin Empire—let's call him Zhang—is far from home, suffering from symptoms that he can't seem to shake. His feet ache and his legs feel weak, sometimes to the point that he can't walk or stand and must lie on his back all day. Worse, he often gets a feeling that there are insects crawling around in his calves, incessantly moving, skittering unpredictably this way and that. Occasionally it's more like alien fingers pinching and kneading him under the skin, climbing up from his calves to his thighs to his belly, higher and higher. It's disconcerting and sometimes debilitating.

Before he came to Jianyang a couple of years ago, Zhang had never experienced such discomforts. He hadn't left Luoyang, his old home in the north, willingly. There'd been no choice; after years of rebellion and strife against the empire, the barbarians had finally succeeded in taking Luoyang—the capital city—along with the emperor himself. They'd killed the crown prince and much of the imperial clan, throwing other aristocratic and official families like his into panic and disarray. Zhang, like many others, had fled far, crossing the mighty Yangzi River and settling here in Jianyang, where a new capital had been established. And so now he resides in the south, a terrifying place so different from the home he'd left, so far from the heartland of classical civilization. The great Chinese empires—the Xia, Shang and Zhou, and the more recent Han—were all governed from the north China plain. Refined culture and virtuous government flourished there, on the dry, silty loess plateau through which the Yellow River rushed. Here, everything is different. The landscape is all curves and hollows, covered in lush green vegetation. There are lakes and streams everywhere, and the soil, too, is damp; mist snakes along the ground. Wild people—are they people?—hide in the hills, speaking incomprehensible tongues and ignorant of the rituals necessary to maintain civilization. And there are beasts, clawed, toothed, and venomous. It is an exile's nightmare.

Zhang knows his condition could be worse: many who've come to this horrible place have contracted sudden turmoil (*huo luan*), with its incessant diarrhea and vomiting, and many have died. Others were felled by cold damage or got *zhang* disease from the misty miasma, alternately shivering and sweating until the miserable end. Some have come down with *gu* illnesses, poisoned by the witchcraft of the local barbarians. So, in comparison, with just leg pains Zhang seems to have escaped the more serious depredations of this toxic environment. Still, he longs to return to health and mobility.

Others in Zhang's social circle have complaints similar to his, and they call their illnesses foot qi. Before they came south they hadn't heard of such a disease, now relatively common. A few healers—a couple of Buddhist monks, some itinerant doctors—are known to be especially good at treating cases of foot qi. Some literate physicians have even put together whole books about it. But what Zhang has found most useful is a little handbook of remedies called *Emergency Formulas to Keep up Your Sleeve*. When Ge Hong, its author, describes foot qi under the heading "Formulas to treat lower leg weakness, numbness, fullness, and rising qi [caused by] wind poison," Zhang recognizes his own condition:

> When one contracts foot qi one is initially unaware. Some feel slight aching or numbness, some have slightly bloated calves, some suddenly feel weak when they start to walk, some lose feeling in the lower abdomen, and some alternate between chills and fever: all these are manifestations.[1]

Then comes the distressing part:

If not promptly treated, [the wind poison] will rise and enter the belly, and its qi will then erupt, thus killing the person.

Perhaps these symptoms are more than the daily annoyance of aches and pains, after all. They require immediate action. Ge Hong recommends drinking fermented soybeans in wine as a prophylactic, and Zhang has begun doing this. He has also followed Ge's advice to burn mugwort leaves at particular points on the body, starting with the neck and moving down to the feet. All of this seems to be having an effect, but the symptoms haven't gone away entirely. Maybe it is time to try Mr. Ge's drug recipes.

* * *

This scenario is imagined, but it is closely based on what early and medieval medical texts tell us about foot qi's origins and symptoms. Evidence suggests that people in China began writing about a disease called foot qi in the late third or early fourth century, that it became visible at a time when the Chinese elite were moving south in large numbers, and that it was considered a disease peculiar to the south, as many other illnesses also were. By examining the earliest written record of foot qi that survives today—Ge Hong's handbook of remedies mentioned earlier—we can glimpse how foot qi was understood in early China and develop a baseline for assessing its transformation in later history. Studying the earliest records of foot qi also provides an opportunity to explore characteristics that foot qi shares with many other early Chinese concepts of illness: it was thought to be caused by an invasion of pernicious qi peculiar to the south and dangerous to particular regional constitutions.

The usual approach to early foot qi is to accept without question the twentieth-century conclusion that everything that goes by this name in historical sources was really the thiamine deficiency disorder beriberi and ask how and when that vitamin deficit can have come about in early China. The historian Peng Wei, for example, points to brief mentions of foot swelling in some of the most ancient Chinese texts—bundles of bamboo and wooden slats created in the third century BC and earlier—as suggestive of thiamine deficiency.

He then seeks to explain how bodies in this period could plausibly have lacked sufficient thiamine: their staple food was rice, steamed in a way that it could have lost vitamin content; there was a lot of infectious disease in this period that could have created the conditions for beriberi to break out.[2] Likewise, H. T. Huang, examining a seventh-century text that says foot qi first emerged in China after the fall of the Han dynasty (third century AD), takes the disease name to indicate beriberi and then tries to explain why thiamine deficiencies suddenly appeared at that time. This leads him to speculate that rice may have been processed differently: "We may presume that pre-Han rice was largely unpolished or lightly polished, while post-Han rice was highly polished, perhaps as highly polished as the rice we are accustomed to seeing today."[3] The presumption is based on the belief that many people were suffering from beriberi, post-Han, not on direct evidence that rice processing technology or behavior had in fact changed.

These are elaborate edifices to build on a rickety foundation, namely the idea that textual mentions of foot qi or foot swelling indicate the presence of beriberi. Approaching early foot qi this way also implicitly belittles the observations and worldview of the people who produced the original texts—celebrating their acumen when they dimly approach modern understandings about diet and disease, and otherwise lamenting their limited knowledge. This chapter and those that follow do not assume that the foot qi premodern doctors were writing about was really the thiamine deficiency disorder beriberi. Instead, they approach the writers' ideas and observations about this disease on their own terms. The aim is to better grasp how Chinese doctors and other intellectuals made sense of illness and healing, rather than subjecting them to what E. P. Thompson called "the enormous condescension of posterity" for not approximating our disease concepts more closely. Here, we learn that the disease name was first used by laypeople and did not appear in the doctrinal classics of Chinese medicine, that it was ambiguous in a way that would allow it to be flexibly applied in different contexts, and that it was marked, from early on, as an ailment specific to northern bodies in the south.

A Humble Beginning: Emergency
Formulas to Keep up Your Sleeve

Generally speaking, the place one wants to begin when telling a story about classical Chinese medicine is the *Yellow Emperor's Inner Canon*. The *Inner Canon* is not the oldest medical text in Chinese; archaeological excavations in recent decades have yielded older examples. But it is the oldest of the texts considered canonical, one that any literate physician in imperial China could be expected to know well. It purports to be a record of exchanges between the Yellow Emperor and his ministers, who initiate their ruler into the arts of healing and maintaining health. It discusses the processes of bodily transformation and illness in abstract, cosmic terms, elaborating concepts that are the foundation of classical Chinese medicine, such as qi, yin and yang, and the five phases, and describing systematic correspondences between changes within the body and changes elsewhere in the natural world. Modern scholars believe that the Yellow Emperor—traditionally dated to the 2600s BC, almost 1,500 years before the earliest Chinese written records—did not actually exist, and that the many short chapters that came to constitute the *Inner Canon* were actually compiled in the third through first centuries BC.[4] Nonetheless, through much of Chinese history the literati considered the *Inner Canon* the cardinal source of authoritative knowledge about maintaining health and grappling with illness.

The term *foot qi* does not appear in the *Inner Canon*, however, so our story cannot begin there. Where, then, should it begin? The fact is that it is impossible to know when, exactly, people in China began to suffer from a disease they labeled foot qi. The earliest written record of the term that we have today dates to the fourth century AD, but, given the relative paucity of sources that have been transmitted from early China, we cannot be sure that it was not written about earlier. Nor does the date of the written sources tell us when people began to *talk* about foot qi; they could have been discussing this category of disease long before anyone decided to write down its name. And in any case, what a fourth-century writer called foot qi might have gone by a different name in earlier medical texts, implying that people had been suffering from these symptoms long before they came to be known by that name. Taking all of that into account, a historian must nevertheless begin where surviving sources do. In the case of foot qi, that means a book called *Emergency Formulas to Keep up Your Sleeve* (*Zhou hou bei ji fang*, hereafter *Emergency Formulas*).[5] It is a book originally written in the early fourth century by Ge Hong, a patrician with many enthusiasms, who came from a district of the Jin empire just south of the Yangzi River. And what it suggests is that foot qi was new, at least in the place where Ge was writing.

The fourth century was a time when the area we now think of as China was politically fragmented. Small states formed, grew, subsumed one another, shrank, and disintegrated in a frequently changing patchwork of territorial control. Modern historians sometimes refer to this as the Period of Division, marking its political fragmentation as an aberration from a presumed norm. This reflects an old prejudice of historians of China, who until recently valorized vast, consolidated empires ruled by a single family and devalued periods between such empires—in this case, between the Han dynasty, which ended in the early third century AD, and the Sui dynasty, which began in the late sixth. "In-between" periods such as this one have suffered undeserved neglect. Scholars have only recently begun to acknowledge that political fragmentation reshaped China in important ways. For example, in the Period of Division the absence of a single powerful government with an official ideology helped foster the rise in China of Buddhism and of Daoist sects, which would influence the literate elite for the rest of imperial history.[6]

Ge Hong thrived in this milieu, and his life and writings reflect the significance of both the state and the new religious landscape in this period. Descended from a clan that had in the past served their state's ruling family, he became a marginal official himself, accepting a series of mostly honorary appointments. These allowed him to pursue his real passion: immortality, which he sought largely by studying alchemy, wandering around the empire in search of the proper setting and ingredients for creating elixirs. He also practiced forms of discipline meant to extend life: physical exercises, patterned breathing, meditation, and prayer. He recorded his techniques for increasing longevity in his best-known work, the *Master Who Embraces Simplicity* (*Bao pu zi*), which later became an important text in the Taiqing tradition of Daoism.[7] Ge's interest in extending life resonates with physicians' interest in preventing death, of course, but the focus on preventing and treating illness in *Emergency Formulas* makes the book unusual in his oeuvre, most of which reflects loftier ambitions. It is not surprising, therefore, that historians of medicine have shown less interest in Ge Hong than have scholars of religion.[8] Besides, historians of early Chinese medicine have paid much more attention to abstract theoretical texts such as the *Inner Canon*. In contrast, humble little formularies or "books of methods" (*fang shu*) such as *Emergency Formulas* focus on the mundane details of treating the sick. Written in a simple, straightforward style, these medical manuals describe patterns of disorder and then recommend appropriate therapies, ranging from drug formulas to dietary changes to physical exercises and moxibustion (a therapy described in the following pages).[9] They specify which drug ingredients can be substituted for others, how many parts herb to how many parts wine one should use, and under what circumstances to increase the dosage of a given drug. The authors who compiled such texts often presented them as a kind of self-help manual for the sick and their caregivers, a handbook of home remedies for people without convenient access to skilled doctors. In the preface to his formulary, Ge declares that his formulas contain "mostly drug ingredients that are easily obtained," and that "those [ingredients] which [patients or their relatives] can't gather and must buy are also all very cheap plants and minerals, found everywhere."[10]

Foot qi's story, then, begins in an unremarkable little book from a relatively neglected historical period. What Ge Hong offers is a layperson's understanding of a set of symptoms and methods for managing them, all attached to a term so general and flexible that it would survive centuries of transformation.

Ambiguity and Flexibility in Early Terms

Ge Hong seems to expect his reader to be familiar with the term foot qi already because he does not provide an etymology, as Chinese writers generally did when introducing new words.[11] Right away, then, we modern readers—who have no such preconceptions or have preconceptions that differ from those of a fourth-century reader—are confronted with ambiguities. First of all, to what does the *qi* in *foot qi* refer? Qi, sometimes written ch'i,[12] is ubiquitous in classical Chinese texts; all material things are made up of it, and it is also the energy or motive force that induces change. The written character depicts steam rising from cooked grain, suggesting vitality, transformation, substance, and nourishment. Nathan Sivin has written:

> By 350 [BC], when philosophy began to be systematic, *ch'i* meant air, breath, vapor, and other pneumatic stuff. It might be congealed or compacted in liquids or solids. *Ch'i* also referred to the balanced and ordered vitalities or energies, partly derived from the air we breathe, that cause physical change and maintain life.[13]

Some scholars have offered English translations such as "configurational energy" or "vital force" or "finest matter influence"[14] for this protean term, but most writing in Western languages today leaves qi untranslated, acknowledging the difficulty of capturing the concept's variety and complexity with one standard term. In a particular context, in one specific usage, one might be able to more accurately capture what an ancient Chinese author meant by *qi*: here, something like energy; here, a kind of illness-causing influence; here, a substance coursing through the body. But the validity of the translation ends at the specific case.

In medicine, doctors distinguished the qi of the body from alien qi from the outside. Bodily qi was the stuff that made up a person—tissues, fluids, and energies that in a healthy person changed and circulated in an orderly, patterned way. Some external qi was essential and could be assimilated into bodily qi. The qi of food and drink, for example, became blood, bones, and sinew once digestive processes had refined it. But the external qi that drew the most medical attention was *xie qi*, sometimes translated as "deviant"—the literal meaning of *xie* being slanted or oblique—"evil," or "heteropathic" qi.[15] This was the wind, the wet, the unseasonable cold or heat that invaded the body and had the potential to wreak havoc. It was the most prominent agent of disorder in Chinese classics. For foot qi, the *xie qi* responsible was wind poison.

Shigehisa Kuriyama has suggested that the prominence of invasive qi in premodern Chinese medicine should make us rethink glib distinctions between a Chinese medicine that focuses on imbalance as a cause of disease and a biomedicine that emphasizes infection. He writes,

> Historically, Chinese doctors saw sickness at least as often in terms of vulnerability and intrusion. Cold and wind attacked, swept in, migrated, bore deeper toward a person's vital core, as if they were discrete entities, grim invaders, disease itself.[16]

This is much like deadly microbes, in other words. However, lest the pendulum swing too far in the other direction, tempting us to anachronistically equate forces like cold and wind with pathogens like bacteria and viruses, it is important to note a couple of ways in which *xie qi* was distinctive. First of all, it was not specific to a disease in the sense that microbes are. The cholera vibrio will produce only cholera, not leprosy or AIDS, but wind poison was implicated not only in foot qi but also in a whole host of otherwise unrelated disorders, from cataracts to sores in the throat to itchy feet and blisters.[17] Also, *xie qi* generally could make a person sick only when combined with an existing vulnerability. If previous illness had weakened the body, excessive emotion had damaged it, or an immoderate lifestyle had destabilized it, then invasive qi might produce symptoms. Otherwise, it posed little threat. Imbalance was thus quite important to Chinese ideas of disease causation, even if no *more* important than invasive qi.

The term *foot qi* is unusual for a Chinese disease name; it blurs the tidy distinction between proper internal qi and deviant external qi. Clearly the qi in the name does not mean *xie qi*, something alien to the body. It seems, instead, to draw attention to the material substance of the feet and legs. But it does not specify the nature of that stuff's dysfunction. Is the qi of the lower legs excessive, deficient, blocked, swelling, reversing, rotting? It is presumably altered in some unhealthy way, but how, exactly, is unclear. This adds to the ambiguity that allows apparently opposite phenomena (lower leg swelling and lower leg shrinking) to be seen as symptoms of the same disease.

Qi is not the only ambiguity here. Even the meaning of *jiao*, which I have translated as "foot," is unclear in Ge's text. It is difficult to know for certain whether *jiao* refers to the feet alone or to the feet and the lower legs. In modern Chinese, *jiao* means "foot," but, according to Zhang Gang, in the period when the earliest references to foot (*jiao*) qi appear, writers used the term *jiao* to indicate everything from the knees down and a more specific term, *zu*, to indicate the foot alone. This usage had already begun to change by the time of Ge's writing, however, with *jiao*'s meaning narrowing to match *zu*'s.[18] Therefore, the *jiao* in *jiao qi* may have already meant "foot" in *Emergency Formulas*. On the other hand, it is also possible that *jiao* retained its older sense in the disease name even after it had come to be synonymous with *zu* in other contexts. The literature makes it clear, after all, that the symptoms of foot qi are not confined to the feet but consistently include the calves and knees as well.

Finally, foot qi is referred to in *Emergency Formulas* as a *bing*. Is this a disease, a disorder, a syndrome? A number of observers today have argued that the focus of classical Chinese medicine was "disorders" or "syndromes" but not "diseases."[19] The word *disorder* connotes a disruption of the body's usual order, of the patterned transformations that define the healthy body. It emphasizes the degree to which each sick person's experience is unique. Because the normal order of one body differs from that of another, two patients' states of disorder may also bear little resemblance to one another. Foot qi *bing*, following this logic, is best translated foot qi disorder, not foot qi disease.

Whether or not today's traditional medicine practitioners think of disease ontologically, however, historically Chinese medical writers have presented some illnesses as more universal than infinitely variable individual experiences. Cold damage diseases, warm diseases, wind diseases, *lai/li* (often translated "leprosy"), flowers of heaven, and foot qi all were written about as objects of study—often the subjects of entire treatises—and as things one could contract. It's true that the wordy title of Ge Hong's section on foot qi evokes variable manifestations ("Formulas to treat lower leg weakness, numbness, fullness, and rising qi [caused by] wind poison") and that one patient's foot qi might manifest quite differently from another's. Still, Ge's discussion begins straightforwardly, "Foot qi *bing* emerged in Lingnan and has spread to Jiangdong."[20] The subject of this sentence is not patients but *bing*; *bing* here seems not only to be abstractable from its sufferers but also mobile, able to spread north from its place of origin. In some contexts identifying the *bing* afflicting a patient was almost as important as identifying what disease a modern patient is suffering from, as a marker of practitioner competence and a way to shape a patient's expectations. Diagnosis—naming the thing afflicting a patient— may not have exercised the same degree of "tyranny" in premodern China as Charles Rosenberg suggests that it does in our time, but it mattered.[21] For this reason, the present book translates *bing* flexibly, depending on context: sometimes "disease" or "diseases," sometimes "disorder" or "disorders."

All this ambiguity may frustrate the modern researcher and reader, but the breadth and flexibility of these words—*jiao, qi, bing*—have helped the term they constitute endure across millennia, find use among both the elite and the ordinary, and embed itself in astonishingly different regimes of knowledge. The term has lent itself to multiple interpretations over time and even to multiple interpretations within a single period, as we shall see.

Northerners in the Toxic South

One of the most conspicuous features of foot qi in *Emergency Formulas* is that it is a regional ailment. It highlights population movement and evolving regional identities. Among the seventy-three categories of illness he addresses, foot qi is the only one for which Ge Hong identifies a region of origin: the south. More specifically, foot qi comes from Lingnan, the area "south of Ling," that is, the Wuling Mountains, which corresponds roughly to Guangzhou and Guangxi provinces in today's China and represented the farthest southern reaches of Chinese empire in Ge's time. Ge believed, however, that the geographical reach of foot qi was growing: it had expanded its range north to

Jiangnan and Jiangdong, the area south and east (*nan* and *dong*) of the Yangzi River (*jiang*).[22] This happened to be Ge's own native place, where he spent most of his life.

Although he associates foot qi with the south, Ge implies that northerners are most vulnerable. At the end of one of his recommended formulas he boasts that "when northerners take this [drug decoction] to treat their feet it is generally effective," as long as high-quality ingredients are used to prepare it. Who were Ge's northerners, and why were they coming into contact with this disease of the south? They were migrants from the north China plain around the Yellow River, refugees who had suddenly inundated the area just south of the Yangzi River where Ge resided. In the past, Chinese empires had been centered on the north China plain, the original heartland of Chinese civilization. Over time, hastened by the ambitions of expansionist governments and by conflict with their northern neighbors, Chinese populations and polities expanded southward. One major spasm of such migration occurred precisely when Ge was writing *Emergency Formulas*. The capital of the Jin empire, the city of Luoyang on the north China plain, had been sacked by rebels in AD 311, and a stream of refugee officials and aristocrats poured south. They crossed the Yangzi River and created a new capital at Jianyang, some thirty kilometers east of Ge's home province. As is often the case during episodes of rapid demographic change, this influx of migrants brought friction and new challenges. Ge himself complained about the dominance of the émigrés and described conflicts between the northern elite and the southerners whose turf they had moved into.[23] Unable to adjust to the new environment, the new arrivals disproportionately fell victim to wind poison and the foot qi it caused.[24]

And no wonder: they encountered a different world from the arid plateau they'd left. The south, with its visible mists wreathing lush hills, its humidity and heavy monsoon rains, seemed to many of them a toxic place with wild beasts, wild people, and an intolerable climate.[25] Mists were miasmas that could make a person sick, and emanations from the moist earth and waterways could invade the body. All of these factors conspired to produce the fatal illnesses common in the region, characterized by vomiting, diarrhea, and intermittent fevers. Northern emigrants considered illness part and parcel of life in the south and a serious impediment to colonization there; in fact, one of the most-discussed southern diseases, *zhang*, was originally written with the same character used to mean "barrier" or "obstruction."[26] To be assigned a post in the far south was often a severe form of exile for errant officials or those on the losing side of factional conflicts in the government—an exile sometimes equivalent to a death sentence.

The toxic south was not thought to imperil those born there to the same degree that it threatened transplants. A person's region of origin shaped his or her constitution, according to the *Yellow Emperor's Inner Canon*, which divided the world into five regions (north, south, east, west, and center) with implications for health and therapy. People from the east, it said, craved salty food and fish and were prone to abscesses; people from the west liked rich food and were vulnerable to internally generated disorder; southerners enjoyed sour and strong-smelling foods and often suffered from cramps and disorders of obstruction; people from the center ate all sorts of things and experienced weakness as one of the main manifestations of illness. Different therapies were also indicated for people from different regions: needling for some; massage, moxibustion, *dao yin* (see Chapter Two), or drugs for others. People from the north, the *Inner Canon* stated, consumed milk and tended to get disorders caused by cold. The full description says:

> In the north is the area where heaven and earth close up and store.
> The land is high, people live in hills, and the wind and cold are freezing. The people there enjoy wild places and eat dairy foods. The cold that they [thus] store up fills them up with disorders. To treat such disorders it is appropriate to use moxibustion, so moxibustion comes from the north.[27]

Moxibustion is a therapy that applies a burning herb, mugwort, on or near particular points on the surface of the body, and its goal is to promote the circulation of qi along fixed channels thought to connect these points with others and with the body's deep interior.[28] Historically, moxibustion developed earlier than acupuncture, though the latter is more widely known and practiced today. Vivienne Lo has argued that, historically, moxibustion and acupuncture were not interchangeable (simply two different ways to stimulate active points, one by burning and one by needling), as they have sometimes been presented. They were thought appropriate for different types of dysfunction, and mugwort for moxibustion was more widely available than fine needles for acupuncture, so moxibustion could be practiced at home by amateurs whereas acupuncture generally required a specialist. The *Inner Canon* is offering a region-based origin story for this staple technique of classical medicine.

The five-part division of regional identity in the *Inner Canon* resonated with the idea of five-phase (*wu xing*) correspondences, the grand unified theory that the early classics synthesized and that later writers preserved and elaborated.[29] According to this theory, every system that exists cycles through a sequence of five states, and the phase of one aspect of the universe (the planets, for example) resonates with and affects the phase of another (a person's body, for instance). Understanding human bodies as falling into five regional types thus allowed physicians and other members of the Chinese literati to integrate a person's region of origin into a coherent, comprehensive matrix that included all features of the natural world: the five flavors, the five seasons, the five musical intonations, and the five sapors of plants and animals used in drug formulas, for example. It made region of origin legible as a data point in the diagnostic and therapeutic process. A patient who was from the west was likely to experience a disorder that had been internally generated, and it was most appropriate to treat that person with toxic drugs.

In practical terms, the regional identities that mattered most were north and south. East, west, and center were necessary to complete the five-phases matrix in a theory-centered text like the *Inner Canon*, but, in more practical genres such as formularies and materia medica, it was northern and southern tendencies that were discussed. Such books emphasized that the different foods and drug ingredients the south produced could upset the orderly functioning of northern bodies, which were more suited to ingesting flora and fauna native to their home region. The eighth-century *Materia Medica for Dietary Therapy*

(*Shi liao ben cao*) by Meng Shen includes careful notes on drug ingredients that were suitable for southerners but not for northerners and vice versa. In the section on seaweed, Meng writes, "Many southerners eat this. They have transmitted [this habit] to northerners. When northerners eat it, it doubly generates the various diseases, and is not suitable for them."[30] Kelp, another form of seaweed, similarly suits southerners but only increases northerners' troubles:

> People on ocean islands are fond of eating kelp. Because they have no good vegetables, they only eat this stuff. They have ingested it for a long time and diseases are not generated. Later, they told northerners about its effectiveness. Northerners ate it, and all the diseases were generated. This is [because] the natural environment did not suit them.[31]

Seaweed, which is perfectly innocuous, or even salutary, in the diets of southerners and islanders, poses a positive health hazard in northern diets, to which it is alien. Similarly, the mutton and milk common to the northern diet were anathema in the south.[32]

Ge Hong seems likewise to recognize that northern constitutions require northern therapies and to subscribe to an understanding of northern affinities similar to the one elaborated in the *Inner Canon* and in Meng Shen's work. Two of his dozen foot qi drug formulas—the ones Ge identifies as particularly effective for northerners—are made with cow's milk, a comestible identified specifically as a northern food in the *Inner Canon*.[33] Ge rarely recommends milk-based remedies in *Emergency Formulas*, so their presence here is notable.

Similarly, moxibustion, the therapy that the *Inner Canon* associates with the north, features prominently among Ge Hong's recommended foot qi treatments, more prominently than in the treatments for any other class of disorder. For other disorders, Ge occasionally recommends burning herbs at a single channel point, slipping the recommendation in between drug formulas and instructions for massage or healing exercises. But for foot qi he lists a whole series of moxibustion formulas, apologizing for not including more:

> The moxibustion methods and channel points [for foot qi] are extremely numerous, [but] I am afraid people [that is, his readers]

cannot completely and precisely know their locations, so here I will only [describe] a few main ones.[34]

He prescribes a series of nine applications of burning herbs, beginning with a point on the spine at the base of the neck and moving down the body to points just above the ankle on the outside of the leg. Because he does not presume that the reader knows the locations of the channel points he names, he adds a description of how to find each. In a typical example, after instructing the reader to burn 100 cones of mugwort at each of the shoulder well points, he explains how to locate the point accurately: "Approach the first sunken place on the shoulders and pinch it with your fingers." To find the wind market point, he suggests standing with arms hanging at the sides and resting one's hands against the outside of the thighs. By twisting the top joint of the middle finger against the thigh where it lies, one can feel the point's location; then one should apply 100 cones of mugwort there. A person who knows little enough about medicine not to know where the channel points lie might be tempted, given that the most prominent symptoms of foot qi are in the lower legs and feet, to try to relieve suffering by burning herbs on these parts of the body. But Ge sternly cautions against this approach, advising, "You must begin from above; if you apply moxibustion to the feet and lower legs straightaway, the qi will rise and not disperse, and [the patient] will consequently be endangered." The great danger in foot qi was rising qi: once the pernicious qi made its way up from the lower extremities to the body's interior, little could be done to save the patient.[35]

Ge's recommendation to use moxibustion not only suggests a regimen tailored to northerners but also emphasizes the importance of treating foot qi when it first appears and the symptoms are relatively superficial—before the qi rises and the disorder becomes acute. Moxibustion seems to have been indicated mostly for yang conditions in Ge's time, in contrast to acupuncture, which seems to have been used on relatively yin conditions.[36] The former manifested in yang parts of the body—the outward surfaces and the extremities—and therefore tended to entail aches, pains, and mechanical dysfunction of various sorts, such as the bloating in the calves or weakness when walking that Ge mentions. Yin conditions emerged from yin areas—generally more internal—and manifested in vomiting, chills and fever, diarrhea, and the like. The prominence of moxibustion among Ge Hong's foot qi remedies, then, suggests the importance of treating foot qi while it still remained a relatively yang condition, before disorder plunged deeper into the body's interior.

This general principle is evident elsewhere in early Chinese medicine, as for example in an incident from the biography of the legendary physician Bian Que, part of the *Records of the Grand Historian* penned by Sima Qian in the early first century BC. Bian Que visits a duke repeatedly, at each visit warning that the duke has an illness and noting that the disorder has moved a little farther toward the interior of the body. The duke, who does not initially feel ill, ignores Bian Que's warnings, and on his last visit, Bian Que abruptly runs out of the audience chamber without so much as a word. Later, questioned about his behavior, Bian Que explains,

> When the disease lies in the pores, it can be treated by poultices.
> When it lies in the blood vessels, it can be treated with needles.
> When it lies in the stomach and intestines, it can be treated with
> medicines. But when the disease lies in the bone marrow, not even
> the God of Life can do anything about it. The duke's disease now lies
> in the bone marrow, and because of this I have no more advice.[37]

The duke, who remains insensible to his own illness until the very end, proves Bian Que's acumen shortly afterward by dying precipitously.

The northerners afflicted with foot qi were powerful aristocrats like the duke, and they apparently regarded their condition with similar insouciance. Like Bian Que, physicians who sought to treat foot qi sufferers were often rebuffed. The initial symptoms—a bit of achiness and numbness, some mild bloating in the calves—must have seemed more nuisance than threat, especially when compared with swiftly deadly disorders such as sudden turmoil or cold damage, which struck occasionally in epidemic form. As Ge indicates, a person first contracting foot qi often does not even perceive it.

Foot qi's initial appearance in writing was not in abstract doctrinal classics but in a formulary written for practical use by someone not formally trained in medicine. The name of the disease itself seems to have been in common use, as Ge's introduction implies. The earliest discussion of foot qi thus reveals how an educated layperson in the fourth century understood this disease and disease more generally— something we can appreciate more when we set aside the false certainty that the disease he was writing about was really a poorly understood vitamin deficiency. Geography was important to Ge, who thought a disease like foot qi could (and had) spread from one region to another. He also thought the same environment had different effects on people from different regions: northern transplants to the south were more vulnerable to foot qi than southerners, even though they breathed the same air, ate the same food, and walked on the same soil. Finally, although the initial effects of foot qi could be subtle, it was insidious and more dangerous than most people realized. By the seventh century, literate physicians began to try to appropriate the common term *foot qi* in their own writings. Unlike Ge Hong, who sought to disseminate medical knowledge to the uninitiated, these physicians attempted to claim knowledge about foot qi as the province of classically educated healers like themselves, recasting some elements of conventional wisdom about it. As we shall see in the next chapter, they were not entirely successful.

CHAPTER TWO

Competing for Medical Authority over Disease

In the early seventh century, the great physician Sun Simiao was called to examine a patient who, having recovered from a previous illness, was now vomiting and weak in the lower legs. After carefully examining the man, Sun announced that he was suffering from foot qi. Sun Simiao, remembered (and sometimes worshiped) by posterity as the "Medicine King," was perhaps the closest approximation in premodern China to a celebrity doctor; he had been invited to serve the emperors of two dynasties and was renowned for his wide learning and clinical virtuosity. He was not the kind of healer whose authority one would expect a layperson to question. In this case, however, his patient demurred. How could it be foot qi, he protested, when he'd never had swollen feet? He refused to take the famous physician's prescription. The patient then turned to other doctors—they suggested that applying a stone needle would cause the deviant qi to dissipate—and paralyzed by indecision over which course of treatment to follow, he ended up dying less than ten days later.[1] Episodes like this one provoked Sun to lament,

> Among the uninitiated there are truly no good doctors. Even if there were, there is rarely a sick person with enough life left in him to enter the care of one. So even when you have a fine steed [that is, an excellent physician], you don't encounter a Bole [a famous judge of fine horses, meaning a patient able to recognize his talent], and even

when you have a Confucius [among doctors], people do not obey him as a teacher deserves.[2]

Sun was hardly the first medical author to complain about the skeptical patient. Throughout imperial history, elite physicians such as Sun Simiao faced diverse and abundant competition for patient patronage. In the *Basic Questions* part of the *Yellow Emperor's Inner Canon*, we find this advice: "Never treat one who is sick but does not approve [your] treatment; treating him will simply be ineffective."[3] And skepticism around foot qi was particularly acute. The disease, with its widely used vague name, tended to strike the rich and powerful and to manifest and remit periodically. This meant that a patient suffering from foot qi was likely to have many different healers at his or her disposal, to consult them repeatedly, and to have his or her own expectations about what foot qi's signs were, as Sun's patient did. Physicians diagnosing foot qi, therefore, often confronted the challenges of the competitive "religio-medical marketplace" of medieval China.[4]

This chapter examines two important medical works of the seventh century to better understand how literate physicians navigated those challenges. The books, *Sources and Symptoms of All Diseases* (*Zhu bing yuan hou lun*) by Chao Yuanfang and *Essential Emergency Formulas Worth a Thousand in Gold* (*Bei ji qian jin yao fang*) by Sun Simiao, addressed an audience of physicians and actively discouraged sick people from treating themselves. Both books questioned what was apparently conventional wisdom about the disease and attempted to present their own knowledge as more authoritative and reliable than the notions of rival healers, patients, and patients' friends and relatives.

In modern discussions of foot qi, and of many other classical Chinese diseases, these two texts are seminal. Those committed to the modern idea that historical foot qi was really the thiamine deficiency disorder beriberi have held up fragments of these texts as important evidence for that identification. In his history of food science in China, for example, H. T. Huang presents the general description of the disease in *Sources and Symptoms* as proof that "the presently understood forms of beriberi . . . were already recognised by the Chinese almost 1,400 years ago."[5] But plucking out the excerpts of physicians' writings that *could* be interpreted as describing a thiamine deficiency diseases does not deepen our understanding of Chinese medicine in this period. Certainly, if it is beriberi you're looking for, you can find it in that excerpt of *Sources and Symptoms*. But those looking for heart disease, heavy metal poisoning, rheumatism, filariasis, or a number of other conditions can equally see them in that same passage, layered as it is with diverse symptoms, none specific to only one modern disease and no single symptom necessary, according to Chao, for a diagnosis of foot qi.[6] Furthermore, the dietary interventions recommended by Sun Simiao, the most renowned physician of his time, are precisely the kind of thing that would exacerbate beriberi: he recommends thiamine-poor polished rice (*jing liang*) and proscribes thiamine-rich animal flesh, including pork.[7] This puts the modern beriberi partisan in the awkward position of suggesting that Sun was unobservant enough to prescribe treatment that would consistently have made his patient sicker. Finally, selectively celebrating the elements of elite doctors' texts that we today see as prescient accepts at face value these doctors' claim that in their own society they were the arbiters of true and false medical knowledge, a claim that their frustrated fulminations belie, as we shall see. This chapter approaches these seventh-century texts with a different aim in mind, looking to them for evidence of how elite physicians defined themselves and their knowledge, how literati doctors' perspectives differed from those of laypeople, and how beliefs about disease were changing. It attempts to illuminate the broader social and cultural context in which the medical authors were working.

Foot Qi for Medical Insiders: Sources and Symptoms of All Diseases

The book that provided the foundation for all later treatises on foot qi was *Sources and Symptoms of All Diseases* (hereafter *Sources and Symptoms*), the grand title of which signals the scope of its ambitions. *Emergency Formulas*, the earlier text examined in Chapter One, had not been seminal when it came to defining the disease. As a kind of home first-aid manual, it offered only the essentials, for quick reference, and seems to have survived mostly because of the fame of its author. In contrast, *Sources and Symptoms* is voluminous and encyclopedic. It was a project commissioned by an emperor and compiled by bureaucrats, and it purported to bring together all that was known about diseases into a single set of volumes. It served as the springboard for virtually all discussions of foot qi in later medieval literature.

The treatise was completed in AD 610, the sixth reign year of the Sui dynasty's second emperor, Yangdi. His family's rule had begun when his father, an energetic duke in one of the many small kingdoms that had proliferated since the collapse of the Han dynasty in the third century, usurped power and established a new state. The former duke then went on to conquer the other small states and reunify the Chinese empire under a single central government. The ambition that had brought about Yangdi's success soon brought about his family's downfall, however. The founding emperor and later his son tried to extend the empire in every direction: south into what is now Vietnam, north into what is now Mongolia, and northeast into what is now Korea. After a series of invasions of the Korean kingdom of Koguryŏ exhausted the treasury and the goodwill of his people, Yangdi's hold on power was tenuous. By the time he died in AD 618, rebellions had sprung up across Sui territory, some led by his own officials and generals. One such insurgent, Yangdi's cousin, succeeded in replacing his regime with a new one that would last centuries longer: the Tang dynasty.

The Sui government's impact, however, was greater than its short duration (AD 581–618) might suggest. Historians writing about this dynasty emphasize its transformative effect on the course of Chinese history. Robert Somers, looking for European analogies, writes, "If the Sui failed to achieve the long period of stable rule we find in major Chinese dynasties, and if they lacked the durability of the Hapsburgs in the West, the regime had the concentrated impact of Europe's Napoleonic era."[8] Likewise, Arthur Wright suggests that without the ambitious emperors of the Sui, the period of disunity in China following the disintegration of the Han might have continued indefinitely. The Sui, he argues, effected the drastic reorganization necessary to prepare the ground for the powerful and long-lived dynasty that succeeded it.[9]

In addition to expanding the empire's territory, Sui emperors also improved its infrastructure, dredging the Grand Canal joining north and south China so that goods and people might pass more easily from one end to the other. They paid attention to ideological consolidation as well, sponsoring new commentaries on all the ancient classics and patronizing Buddhist, Daoist, and Confucian scholars. Civil engineering and cultural projects thus took their places alongside military adventurism as part of a larger effort to build a strong, unified empire. *Sources and Symptoms* typifies this broader unifying effort. At Yangdi's behest, the medical official Chao Yuanfang and his mostly unnamed assistants created a textbook intended to order then-current knowledge about disease and standardize the training of imperial medical staff.

Chao Yuanfang was an erudite for general medicine in the Imperial Medical Office.[10] One source reports that Chao successfully treated a senior military commander for a wind reversing disease that had him bedridden. "I have not yet finished the prescription yet I have completely recovered!" the commander exclaimed. Not long afterwards, the emperor made Chao chief editor of the disease project, apparently impressed by his skill in diagnosis and treatment.[11] His official title signals one of the changes in the institutionalization of medicine that began in this period. The position of medical erudite had no equivalent in the government of the Han dynasty (206 BC–AD 220), the earliest long-lasting bureaucratic empire in China. The Han government had employed three learned physicians: one who diagnosed and prescribed for palace residents, one responsible for securing and maintaining drug ingredients, and one responsible for compounding prescriptions. But the Han government had no offices charged with writing, compiling, and revising medical texts. The Sui government, basing its medical bureaucracy on what the northern dynasties had developed during the Period of Division, not only expanded the number of medical personnel (physicians, pharmacists, and even incantation and talisman-making experts) working for the emperor and his family to include more than seventy but also added an Imperial Medical Office that trained students and produced authoritative texts. *Sources and Symptoms* thus was a kind of textbook for a newly enlarged school for physicians—not only doctors to the imperial household but all of those employed in government service. In both ideological and practical senses, it is appropriate to see *Sources and Symptoms* as a project characteristic of imperial ambitions, at once asserting state authority over a comprehensive body of knowledge, and helping to expand a medical bureaucracy.

As befits a textbook for government physicians, *Sources and Symptoms* is clearly meant for an audience with medical expertise. It assumes that the reader knows how to feel and evaluate the pulse, for example, specifying that foot qi sufferers have three characteristic pulses: "floating, large, and slack"; "rapid and tight"; and "slight and feeble."[12] The art of pulse diagnosis was vitally important to early learned medicine in China,[13] and it bore little resemblance to pulse taking in today's biomedicine, in which doctors focus almost exclusively on the rapidity and regularity of the heartbeat. Doctors trained in classical Chinese medicine—like Western doctors before the nineteenth century, for that matter[14]—attuned themselves to more subjective aspects of what they felt under their fingers. Placing three fingers against the underside of the forearm just below the wrist, they felt the pulse at three depths, first lightly at the surface, then pressing a bit deeper, and finally feeling the deep pulse with even more pressure. They used terms such as floating, sinking, full, shrunken, taut, slack, and many more to describe the sensations and sometimes illustrated them with drawings meant to capture and convey the feeling associated with those descriptors (see Figure 1). The doctor's evaluation was thus, to a large degree, embodied—that is, contained in his own bodily sensations. When diagnosing, he assessed both his own and the patient's experience of the patient's condition.[15]

For an experienced physician, then, *Sources and Symptoms*'s brisk invocation of foot qi pulse sensations would have been perfectly comprehensible:

> If the patient's pulse is floating, large, and slack, you can administer two doses of Continuing-Life Decoction. If wind [poison] is abundant then it is suitable to give Maidservant from Yue Decoction and add four *liang* [about 53 grams] of *Atractylodes* [*zhu*] to treat it. If the pulse turns rapid and tight, you should give Bamboo Sap Decoction.

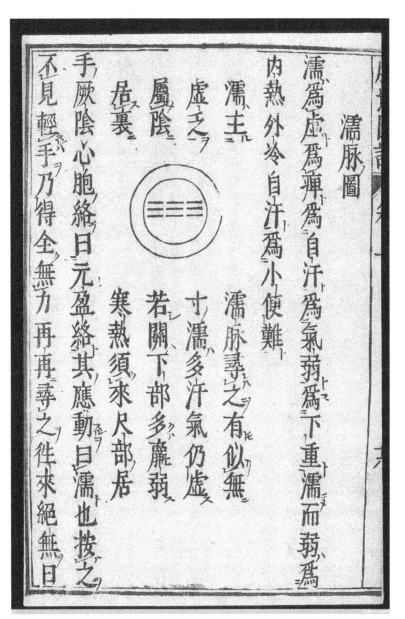

濡脈圖

濡為虛為痺為自汗為氣弱為下重濡而弱為
內熱外冷自汗為小便難
濡主
虛乏
屬陰
居裏
濡脈尋之有似無
寸濡多汗氣仍虛
若關下部多癃弱
寒熱須來尺部居
手厥陰心胞絡曰元盈絡其應動曰濡也按之
不見輕手乃得全無力再再尋之往來絕無曰

FIGURE 1. Illustration of "Soggy Pulse (*rumai*)," from *Ren yuan mai ying
gui zhi tu shuo* (Pictorial Handbook of Pulse Images Based on the Person),
attributed to Wang Shuhe (third century AD) and revised by Shen Jifen between
the fourteenth and seventeenth centuries. The text states, in part: "Soggy
Pulse . . . is imperceptible when pressed and can be felt only with a gentle
touch; it lacks force and feels like cotton floating in water."

If the pulse is slight and feeble, you should give two to three doses of Wind-Drawing Decoction . . . If the patient is greatly depleted and short of breath, you can administer tonifying medicines during this time, according to the heat or coldness of the sick [person's] body. If the patient still is not cured, make some more Bamboo Sap Decoction . . . you must use your perception and accord with the situation.[16]

To laypeople, however, the diagnostic and therapeutic instructions above must have seemed nearly as cryptic as they are to a modern reader. Not only does the author assume that his reader can distinguish among different pulses (for all of which, he states, the external symptoms may be the same), he also expects that reader to know how to create Continuing-Life Decoction, Maidservant from Yue Decoction, Bamboo Sap Decoction, and Wind-Drawing Decoction, as he invokes the names of these formulas without offering instructions for making them. A basic understanding of how to make a decoction— that is, a liquid medicine prepared by boiling plants and sometimes minerals and animal parts—was probably widespread. And it would have been possible, perhaps, to excavate the ingredients and treatment rationale from formularies circulating at the time; contemporary reference works based on premodern formularies suggest that ephedra (*ma huang*), licorice root (*gan cao*), rhizome of *chuan xiong*, root of *fang feng*, ginger root, scutellaria (*huang qin*), and ginseng (*ren shen*), consistently featured in the named formulas, were meant to disperse wind, induce sweating, clear heat, move water, and support the circulation of normal qi.[17] But the reference works mentioned, each many hundreds of pages long, also give a sense of the volume of relevant knowledge underlying the simple shorthand of something like "Continuing-Life Decoction." To know which ingredients to use and how to compound these named decoctions, one would have needed either to have access to multiple formularies or to have received instruction in pharmacology.

The only therapeutic techniques that the book elaborates on are *yang sheng* and *dao yin* techniques. *Yang sheng* or "nurturing life" practices aimed to fortify the body and prevent illness, something the earliest medical classics had promoted as superior to healing.[18] As the

Inner Canon famously declares, seeking treatment when illness has already developed is like digging a well when one feels thirsty or casting weapons after a battle has started—an example of taking action too late. Far better to "put in order what [is] not yet in disorder" by engaging in disciplined movement and breathing and arranging one's sleep, work, sexual activity, emotions, and diet to accord with the season and with one's phase of life.[19] Even in a threatening natural environment, surrounded by noxious qi, the person who has thus cultivated a robust constitution need not fear that she will fall ill. Wind poison, wet and cold, miasmic qi: all require a preexisting vulnerability, the *xu* or systemic depletion of a body inadequately cared for, before they can invade and wreak havoc.[20] Of course, as a manual devoted to disease, *Sources and Symptoms* primarily teaches treatment, not prevention. Nevertheless, it does identify some appropriate *yang sheng-dao yin* techniques, perhaps for those who have managed to recover from an illness and want to avoid a relapse.

Dao yin can be translated literally as "guiding and pulling." *Dao* means to guide or direct, in this case guiding qi around and out of the body. *Yin* in its original meaning indicated pulling taut a bowstring to shoot an arrow, and in its more abstract sense it suggests "the pulling and activating of strength and inner tension," as Livia Kohn phrases it.[21] In the past, *dao yin* has sometimes been translated "gymnastics," but the English word's association with performative athleticism (at least, in the United States) has led scholars such as Kohn to reject this translation and to propose "healing exercises" as a more accurate reflection of what it connotes.[22]

Sources and Symptoms recommends five exercises for foot qi that it identifies as "*yang sheng* formulas and *dao yin* methods." Here is a typical example:

Bend one foot, toes facing upward. Tighten [your body]. Press one foot against the kneecap. Then relax your mind and expel *qi* downward from the ankles. With one hand knead the kneecap and press down forcefully. Place the other hand in back and knead the mat. After a while, straighten out. Do both the right and left this way, fourteen [times]. This gets rid of acute soreness in the knee and thigh.[23]

The other exercises similarly combine mental relaxation with expelling qi downward (countering the dangerous qi's tendency to rise, which we have seen is how foot qi characteristically develops) and stretching, tightening, and kneading the knees and feet. Every description ends with the promise that the exercise described will eliminate some of foot qi's painful manifestations: lower leg aching and weakness, tautness and pain in the calves, cold in the knees, cramps, and the other "gradual daily depredations." Nowhere does the author suggest that the *dao yin* exercises will cure foot qi; they will not, by themselves, expel the wind poison from the system. Rather, they aim at managing the disease's effects.

Although the mechanics of these exercises are described clearly, unlike the drug formulas named earlier, they too assume a certain amount of medical knowledge. Two of them instruct the afflicted person to make use of a particular channel point—in one, the *yong quan* point and in the other the *jie xi* point—either circulating qi toward it or pressing on it. Without either specialized training or access to technical reference works, the reader would have been unlikely to know that the *yong quan* point lay slightly forward of the center of the sole, or that the *jie xi* point was located at the crease where the front part of the foot meets the lower leg.[24]

In short, although *Sources and Symptoms* does not explicitly disparage those without medical training, it makes no effort to include them, either. The anticipated reader is one well versed in the locations of channel points, the recipes for drug formulas, and subtle differences in the sensations that pulses present to experienced fingers.

The Celebrity Physician and His Rivals

The other major work to discuss foot qi diseases and their clinical challenges in this period was Sun Simiao's *Formulas Worth a Thousand in Gold*. We met Sun at the beginning of the chapter, a learned scholar and skilled physician who outlived the Sui dynasty and then saw some six decades of the Tang. Like Ge Hong, the centuries-earlier author of *Emergency Formulas to Keep up Your Sleeve*, Sun pursued longevity through alchemy, but unlike Ge his vocation was that of a physician. He spent most of his life treating patients in north China and spent his last years in the mountains of what is now Shaanxi province, expanding his knowledge of medicinal herbs. His medical works are therefore more widely remembered and read than his alchemical treatise. And although he attracted the attention of emperors, Sun refused their repeated invitations to enter government service.[25] In contrast to Chao Yuanfang, then, Sun did not produce *Formulas Worth a Thousand in Gold* at the behest of a central government, and he was not helped in his efforts by an editorial staff.

There are many reasons for the lasting influence of *Formulas Worth a Thousand in Gold*. It is considered the first Chinese book to address medical ethics; the section called "The Perfect Integrity of the Great Physician" (*da yi jing cheng*) is frequently cited as a kind of Chinese Hippocratic Oath.[26] In addition, the book's extensive treatment of diseases specific to women made it the touchstone of gynecological literature in later centuries and has drawn the attention of historians curious about the experiences of women in imperial China.[27] *Formulas Worth a Thousand in Gold* synthesizes and preserves material from an impressively wide range of sources. With only one major exception, Sun seems to draw on all the earlier medical works available to us today and more.[28] Small wonder that the book is integral to the classical medical canon, to the extent that it is still used in Traditional Chinese Medicine curricula in China today.

Like *Sources and Symptoms*, *Formulas Worth a Thousand* is clinical in its orientation; its primary audience seems to be physicians rather than laypeople. The chapter on foot qi takes clinical puzzles as the basis for organization, as a sampling of its section headings indicates: "On why [foot qi diseases] are contracted in the feet," "On diseases that recur because [a patient has] foot qi," "On whether [foot qi diseases are caused by] depletion or repletion; drugs you can administer, and drugs you cannot," and "On how one can cure those amenable to treatment in several days." These are clearly aimed at the practicing physician rather than the suffering patient or her caregivers.

In fact, as Sun depicts them, those without medical training are meddlesome and ignorant, however well meaning they may be. One section of his foot qi chapter is titled "On people who visit the sick to ask after their illness," and in it he excoriates such busybodies:

> These people have not experienced a single thing. They have never read one single formula. They show off [as if they] understand completely, and falsely make themselves out to be perspicacious and skilled. When they talk [about the illness] they come to different conclusions. Sometimes they say, "This is depletion," sometimes they say, "this is repletion." Sometimes they say, "This is wind," sometimes they say, "This is *gu* [a kind of witchcraft then associated with southern regions]." Sometimes they say, "This is water," sometimes they say, "This is phlegm." They speak recklessly and erroneously, and each kind [of error] is different. [This] wrecks the sick person's mind and will; he doesn't know what is true, and vacillates and doesn't make a decision. Time does not wait for people. When [their advice] suddenly brings about disaster, each [of the advice-givers] naturally scatters and departs. This is why there is a great need for good people and good, renowned doctors to see patients—ones who can distinguish shallow from deep disorder, who have investigated formularies, who have read widely in ancient and modern [texts], who can clearly explain every [illness] episode. Otherwise, people's affairs will be greatly harmed.[29]

Sun vividly expresses what was a general problem for physicians in premodern China. Unlike rich industrialized societies today, where biomedicine has more cultural and social authority than any other form of healing, in imperial China physicians like Sun who were educated in medical classics did not automatically have more credibility than their competitors. No guilds or state certification existed to restrict entry into the society of healers. Sick people embraced a wide range of healing beliefs and practices, and there was no general prejudice favoring elite healers like Sun Simiao—the literati physicians known as *yi*—as more efficacious than others. In fact, if anything, the prevailing prejudice worked against them. It was not unusual for a patient to reject the advice of an elite physician and embrace the treatment of a less educated but more trusted healer instead. Evidence suggests that most people in early and medieval China did not generally think of disease as a natural phenomenon to be treated by natural means but as an affliction brought on by spirits, best treated by ritual specialists of one sort or another. Nathan Sivin has argued for the eleventh century—and it is likely to have been true many centuries earlier—that sick people sought help from popular priests, Buddhists, and Daoists, in descending order of frequency. Very few had access to literati physicians such as Sun, and even they did not hesitate to also consult midwives, spirit mediums, bonesetters, nuns and priests, and hereditary herbalists.[30]

Nor was the treatment of illness the only arena in which physicians found themselves challenged by other claimants to authority. The same Sui and Tang elite who sought out physicians for "nurturing life" (*yang sheng*) advice also patronized the diverse forms of vitality- and longevity-boosting that the Daoists had developed—sometimes sampling them a bit too liberally. Six Tang emperors are said to have died from elixir poisoning brought on by formulas meant to make them immortal. Perhaps surprisingly, such deaths did not necessarily discredit Daoist immortality elixirs because—especially in a society where Buddhist ideas of the cycle of rebirth and suffering were prevalent—death "could be interpreted as successful metamorphosis and release from the world."[31] This gives a sense of how pluralistic the views of the elite were at this time.

What did it mean to be a literati physician in this cosmopolitan society, with its diverse sources of healing? Sun Simiao offers some idea when he elaborates on his definition of "good, renowned doctors": one of their most important traits is that they have "investigated books of methods" and have "read widely in ancient and modern [texts]." Since at least the third century BC, the training of *yi* had revolved around texts and in general required formal initiation into a text-owning lineage. At a time when all books were handwritten manuscripts, they were few, precious, and jealously guarded. A prospective pupil, accordingly, had to prove his moral and intellectual worth before a teacher would agree to share such a treasure. Only after the apprentice had demonstrated that he was one of the "right people" (*qi ren*) who could be trusted to preserve the reputation of the lineage was he formally admitted and allowed to receive the master's texts, a moment that might be marked by a blood oath emphasizing the new physician's duty not to transmit them to the unworthy.[32] In later centuries, when the spread of printing and publishing made books more widely available, it would become possible to be a medical autodidact, to read a few books by famous physicians and count oneself their disciple. But in this period, an aspiring *yi* obtained the manuscript in an intimate face-to-face setting, only after sustained effort.

Once initiated into a lineage, the newly minted doctor could trade on its reputation to attract the patronage of the well-heeled and powerful. In the period in which Sun Simiao was writing, however, the pool of potential clients shrank a bit as compared with the preceding centuries. When small states dominated the political map between the third and sixth centuries, there had been many different loci of power, and aristocratic families in the various states had flourished. Once the Sui and Tang governments reunified China, however, their ruling families quickly sought to eliminate rivals, weakening other aristocratic families through legal changes and by promoting the civil service examination system, formerly a minor adjunct to a recommendation-fueled system, as a means to official appointment. For physicians this meant fewer families with the status and wealth to keep an elite physician on retainer.[33] The desire to attract the eminent patrons who remained, and to attract able disciples to ensure the continued eminence of one's lineage, likely motivated *yi* to explicitly contrast their skill with competitors.

In addition, the form of medical literature had changed. Earlier, the texts transmitted within literati lineages had tended, like the *Inner Canon*, to be attributed to divine or legendary figures and to take the form of dialogues between those legendary figures and their initiates (or initiators; sometimes the roles are reversed). But whereas earlier texts had obscured their authorship and derived their authority from association with divine figures, starting in the second century AD medical writers had begun to identify themselves as the authors and even to include prefaces indicating their motivation for writing.[34] The age of celebrity medical authors had begun; producing texts helped generate and maintain a reputation in a way that had not been possible before. There was a more natural place in this sort of writing for complaints about ignorant rivals and bullheaded patients than there had been in the earlier conversations-with-immortals genre. Thus the frictions of practicing in a competitive environment, and alternative understandings of disease, are more visible in the texts of this period than they had been before.

Trust Me, I'm a Doctor: Literate Physicians Appropriate Foot Qi

Seventh-century sources on foot qi betray the irritation some elite physicians felt when patients rejected their judgments. The question of how to diagnose and treat this disease seems to have provoked particular debate within the menagerie of healers, patients, and caregivers. Its name had apparently come from popular usage, rather than from the sophisticated texts of correlative cosmology that underlay learned medicine. What's more, some of the earliest experts on foot qi had been Buddhist monks.[35] Even patients themselves, with no claim to any healing tradition, thought they understood the nature of foot qi quite well. These realities made it especially difficult for literati doctors to claim any kind of exclusive expertise in this area.

That doesn't mean they didn't try, however. Both *Sources and Symptoms* and *Formulas Worth a Thousand in Gold* attempt to dispel common beliefs about foot qi, and both insist that their authors' approach, based on the principles and skills of classical medicine, is the correct one. One of the most dangerous misconceptions, they suggest, is that foot qi is minor and not urgent. *Sources and Symptoms* ominously stresses how insidious it is:

> When they get this illness, most people do not immediately feel it. Some first have no other disease and then suddenly get [this one]; some contract it after suffering multiple other illnesses. In the beginning the symptoms are trivial; [the patient] eats, drinks, and amuses himself the same as ever, and his physical strength is the same as before. At this time one must observe [the condition] carefully.[36]

If, lulled into complacency by the seemingly trivial initial symptoms, a person fails to call a doctor, the pernicious qi proceeds upward toward the belly and chest and precipitates a fatal crisis. Chao writes, "If one is slow to treat [this illness], it easily rises and enters the belly. When it has entered the belly . . . [and] the chest and flank fill up and the qi rises, it can easily kill a person. The acutely ill will not live out the day; the less ill sometimes have one to three days."[37] Sun agrees that foot qi can kill, innocuous though it may appear at first, and suggests that prompt, competent care is required to manage it. He classes those who die needlessly of foot qi in three categories: the ones who perceive the illness too late to treat it, the ones who are too proud to seek a doctor for such an apparently minor complaint, and the ones who agonize by themselves and can't decide what to do.[38] Other seventh-century physicians echoed the warning against approaching foot qi too cavalierly. Su Jing, the author of *Treatise on Foot Qi* (*Jiao qi lun*), stated categorically, "Foot qi is not fatal; if you won't accept treatment, you are bringing death upon yourself, that is all. It is not the disease that kills people," but refusing to seek timely treatment.[39]

As we saw at the beginning of the chapter, one common belief about foot qi was that swelling of the feet was its signal symptom. Not so, Sun asserts. It may be a common manifestation, but "One should not think of swelling as a symptom of foot qi in every case. There are those that [involve] swelling, [but] there are also those that do not [involve] swelling."[40] *Sources and Symptoms* concurs, saying that foot qi's first outward manifestations are indeed in the lower legs but are not necessarily swelling. Instead, the consistent initial symptom is "numbness from the knees to the feet." Other signs vary enormously:

> Sometimes there is aching, sometimes a creeping sensation like insects crawling around. In some cases the area from the toes to the knee and calf is especially sensitive to cold. In some cases the lower leg is bent and weak and [the patient] cannot walk. In some cases the lower legs have slight swelling, extreme sensitivity to cold, or pain. In some cases [the lower legs] are relaxed and do not obey [the patient's intentions], or are convulsed. There are some whose condition is dire [yet] they can still eat and drink; [but] some cannot. Some vomit upon seeing food and drink, and can't stand the smell of food. There are those who feel a thing like fingers, dispatched from the meaty

part of the calf, which travel upward and attack the heart, and the qi
rises. Some have spasms over the entire body. Some have serious hot
sensations and headache. Some people's chests and hearts rush and
throb [as though frightened], and they cannot stand to see light in
the places where they sleep. Some patients have a bitter pain in their
bellies and simultaneous diarrhea; in some, their language is confused
and they easily forget or mistake things. Some have blurred vision
and mental confusion. All of these are signs of the illness.

Here, the writers subsume what some understand to be the major
sign of foot qi, swelling in the lower legs, in a much longer litany of
possible signs. Clearly, they imply, foot qi is not so simple to identify.

What about the idea, reflected in earlier mentions of foot qi in
laypeople's formularies, that it is caused by wind poison and exclusive to the south? Sun and the authors of *Sources and Symptoms* agree
that wind poison in the environment is the causative qi. *Sources and
Symptoms* states categorically that "all foot qi disease is incurred by
contracting wind poison."[41] For his part, Sun describes in more detail
how such poison enters the body: "All wind-poison qi rises from the
ground. The cold, heat, wind and wet of the earth all produce vapor-
ous qi, and the feet frequently tread on [the earth], so when wind
poison attacks a person, it always first attacks the lower legs."[42] Accordingly, he offers a sensible precaution:

> Do not stand or sit in cold, wet places for long periods . . . if in the
> summer months you sit or stand for a long time on wet ground, then
> hot, wet qi will steam up into your circulation tracts . . . if in the
> winter months you sit or stand on wet, cold ground for a long time,
> then cold, wet qi will rise and enter your circulation tracts.[43]

Where Sun differs with *Sources and Symptoms*, however, is in identifying wind poison's geographical limits. *Sources and Symptoms*, like Ge
Hong's *Emergency Formulas* three centuries earlier, indicates the same
area south of the Yangzi River as the hotspot: "In Jiangdong and Lingnan, the land lies low, and wind and wet qi can easily harm people."[44]
Sun Simiao, however, disagrees with *Sources and Symptoms* that foot
qi is exclusive to the steamy south. He argues that one can contract it
anywhere. This has not always been true, he concedes: in the time of

the Three Kingdoms (ca. AD 200 to 280), the disease was unknown in the north. But now people all over the empire experience it.

What changed? Back in the third century, Sun explains, "Customs and teachings were not yet unified, frost and dew were uneven, and cold and heat were unequal [in different parts of China]. Thus west of the mountain passes and north of the Yellow River, this disease was unknown." Here he suggests that in that time of political disunity, not only did education and customs differ from one part of China to another, but the characteristic qi of the natural environment did too: some places were cold, with abundant frost, whereas others were hot, and morning dew was more common. But Sun continues,

> Ever since the current emperor's expansion [of territory], no place falls outside the empire in any direction . . . lately, even when the gentry of the Middle Kingdom do not cross south of the Yangzi River, there are unexpectedly also those among them who suffer this illness. This comes about because today the wind qi of every place under heaven is mixed together.[45]

In other words, wind poison is not a static feature of a landscape for Sun. It can appear where it has not existed before; political consolidation spreads environmental qi and makes it uniform, just as it spreads human institutions and infrastructure.

But what was the mechanism? How did diverse environments homogenize, mixing together the "wind qi of every place under heaven"? Did the large numbers of people moving across the newly consolidated empire—soldiers deployed to pacify the south, officials appointed to posts distant from their native places, merchants taking advantage of improved roads and canals to extend their trading routes—carry wind poison with them? Did Sun think of wind qi as stowing away in their bodies as we now think the smallpox virus did in sixteenth-century Europeans traversing the Atlantic, or the plague bacillus did in fleas that moved across Central Asia with the Mongols in the thirteenth century? Precautions Chinese people took during epidemics suggest that they did sometimes believe people and objects could harbor disease.[46] Still, it is unlikely that Sun had in mind a concept of contagion like the one that informs our modern understanding of the Black Death or the depopulation of the Americas. He probably did not conceive of wind qi as something that was schlepped, wittingly or not, by physical bodies across space. More likely, he conceived of environmental features such as heat, cold, and wind qi as responding in a more abstract way to vigorous government; this is consistent with many centuries of Chinese thought about resonance effecting change. According to the *Analects* of Confucius, for example, a good ruler exerts influence through his own virtuous example rather than laws and punishments, and the people align themselves with his will unconsciously, as grass bends before the wind or lesser stars rotate around the North Star.[47] As the later Confucian philosopher Mencius put it, when one possesses the appropriate virtue, governing the world is "as easy a matter as to make anything go round in the palm."[48] Similarly, alchemists, among whom Sun can be counted, thought successfully creating an elixir required recapitulating in reverse the orderly development of the cosmos, not merely inducing particular chemical reactions and mechanical changes in the substances themselves.[49] In many of the classics, social and material conditions change because things resonate spontaneously with a new order that has developed in the system of which they are a part. So might the qi of diverse regions have homogenized spontaneously under the new order that the Tang government brought to all under heaven. Sun's belief that China's environment changed over time accords with what modern paleoclimatologists tell us; north China was affected, like the rest of the world, by a global cooling in the early centuries AD, a Medieval Warm period peaking in the 1200s, and a Little Ice Age between 1400 and 1800.[50] But unlike modern scientists, Sun saw human activity—political change—as the primary stimulus for premodern environmental changes that had an impact on health.

Although they disagree about whether foot qi is confined to the south, the seventh-century sources agree that, pace Ge Hong, northerners are not particularly prone to it. Neither *Sources and Symptoms* nor *Formulas Worth a Thousand in Gold* mentions northerners, and neither especially recommends moxibustion or milk—therapies that the *Inner Canon* had associated with northern constitutions—as treatments. These differences might indicate that foot qi had become more common in Jiangdong than it had been three centuries earlier or that Chao and Sun, being themselves what Ge Hong would have called northerners, did not think of "northerner" as a marked, distinctive identity. In their world, those contracting the disease were not an intrusive group of outsiders, but people like themselves.

Instead of northern origins, the seventh-century sources identify a different attribute that renders a person vulnerable to foot qi: plumpness. *Sources and Symptoms* suggests that it was the "spaces in the skin of plump people" that allowed pernicious qi, steaming up from the damp ground, to invade.[51] Sun Simiao writes that people

> who are dark [that is, have dark complexions] and skinny are easy to treat; those with a lot of fat, thick flesh, and red and white [complexions] are hard to cure. Dark-complected people can tolerate wind and wet [qi], [but] red-and-white-complected people do not tolerate wind. The flesh of skinny people is hard, and of fat people is soft. When the flesh is soft [as in fat people] the disease penetrates deeply.[52]

This observation leads Sun to warn against using tonifying therapies, those meant to stimulate and strengthen the patient's own bodily qi. "In all cases," he cautions, "[it is] from repletion of qi that one dies." Therefore, the most appropriate treatment is depleting drugs, those that attenuate the sick body's own tendency toward repletion:

> There has never been a single person who has taken medicine [for foot qi] to bring about depletion and died. Therefore people who have foot qi should not take powerful tonics, and also should not take powerful purgatives, and finally should not fear depletion and for that reason stop a decoction early, refusing to take it. Those who do such things will all die and you should not treat them.[53]

In this regard, foot qi subverted the usual expectations of classical Chinese medicine, which tended to focus on the dangers of depletion (*xu*)—"a pathology of dissipation," as Kuriyama puts it—rather than repletion (*shi*).[54] Early Chinese physicians thought the depleted body invited illness, being unable to fight off invasive qi from the outside. Many drugs, as well as techniques such as needling, were therefore intended to strengthen the body to help it resist and expel such unwelcome forces. If a person believed, as all these early sources agree, that invading wind poison caused foot qi, the disease would seem to be a prime example of how depletion might leave one vulnerable—and one can understand why, in the consultation described at the beginning of this chapter, Sun's rivals prescribed applying stone needles. But Sun bucks the conventional wisdom, asserting that in these illnesses, it is excess, not deficiency, that kills. Wind qi might invade any body type, but skinny bodies prone to depletion resisted the internal movement of wind and wet qi fairly well, whereas fat, ruddy ones allowed it to sink in.

Moreover, Sun's list of foods that foot qi sufferers should avoid—mutton, beef, fish, butter, pork, chicken, goose, duck, and more—suggests patients whose regular diet did not lack in variety and abundance. Meat was such a luxury that the vast majority of the population generally ate it only once a year during the New Year festival and at the occasional community sacrificial ritual, if ever. Even officials, sometimes called "meat-eaters" to highlight their privilege, probably did not actually eat meat very often.[55] To proscribe meats, then, would only have been meaningful for an exceptionally well-off segment of the population. In that light, Sun's insistence that repletion, rather than depletion, fostered foot qi seems almost commonsensical.

Both of these important sources aimed to reach physicians and to convince them that what patients, patients' relatives, and perhaps physician-readers themselves believed about foot qi was mistaken. Sun, in particular, seems troubled by rival healers and skeptical patients. He complains repeatedly about their misconceptions and sighs ostentatiously over the damage they wreak, framing much of his discussion in the negative: what not to believe, how not to proceed, how others fail. *Sources and Symptoms*, by contrast, does not explicitly malign ignorant physicians or laypeople. Perhaps this is because Chao and his team, as government functionaries, had the security of their sinecures to comfort them and did not have a reputation such as Sun's to maintain. But *Sources and Symptoms* does emphasize the complexity and danger of foot qi, implying that people do not take it seriously enough.

Taken together, these sources reflect the medical marketplace in which their authors lived, in which even a very educated physician, with lofty official connections, faced skepticism from patients and competition from rivals. They reflect, moreover, the social significance of a foot qi diagnosis in medieval Chinese society. As an affliction that particularly vexed the elite, developed gradually, and needed to be managed over a span of years or even decades, foot qi promised a lucrative and long-lasting source of patronage for the healer who managed to install himself as the sufferer's first choice. The opportunity they presented to healers, therefore, was greater than that created by epidemic diseases that killed quickly and felled poor and rich in equal proportion. Rhetoric disparaging rivals was correspondingly sharp. Illuminating the tensions in seventh-century writings about foot qi thus helps us to better appreciate the social, political, and economic circumstances that shaped perceptions of disease. Clearly laypeople had their own understandings of foot qi that differed from those of elite physicians; to the extent that we can excavate them, should those concepts be any less a part of its history?

Previous histories have presumed that the most important thing one can learn from these texts is, as the historian Fan Ka-Wai puts it, the "disease to which [foot qi] corresponds according to modern medical concepts."[56] Some, ignoring complicating evidence, assert that that disease was unambiguously beriberi. Other studies consider the symptoms described and conclude that seventh-century foot qi must have been something else.[57] But all alike privilege modern disease definitions as the last word, as though the primary task of historical research on disease should be to extract nuggets of empirical observation from the tailings of fallacious theory. Historical doctors' own interpretations, when they are considered at all, are assessed according to how closely they resemble the modern understanding. Thus, elite doctors earn points for occasionally expressing an opinion such as "prolonged consumption of rice weakens the body," or suggesting a single remedy that contains substantial thiamine. When they fail to elevate those ideas and remedies to central importance, the modern chronicler cries out in disappointment.[58]

Such scoring of healers by the standards of modern knowledge tells us little of interest about seventh-century Chinese medicine. No one will get a perfect score because no one in the seventh century came up with the idea that eating too little vitamin B can kill a person. And training our eyes on the scorecard keeps us from appreciating the interesting things that they noticed and caring about the conclusions they drew: how political change seemed to impact public health, for example, and how complexion and body type seemed to be correlated with a particular kind of illness. It prevents us from more fully understanding the medical world they inhabited, how they fashioned their authority and shored up their credibility.

Developments in the tenth through thirteenth centuries ensured that foot qi—its proper diagnosis and treatment—would remain actively contested through the end of imperial history, as the next chapter shows. In that period, printing technology combined with new governmental aspirations and the resulting literature further complicated China's competitive healing environment. It also, however, yielded concepts that unlike most in premodern medicine would eventually be incorporated into modern biomedicine.

CHAPTER THREE

Simplifying and Standardizing Disease

In the centuries after Sun Simiao lamented the general state of igno-rance about foot qi, it continued to nettle elite physicians who saw it as misunderstood and incompetently treated. In the thirteenth cen-tury the eminent Zhang Congzheng (ca. 1156–1228) grumbled that when it came to so-called foot qi, patients and their caregivers tried all sorts of therapies unmoored from any underlying principle: "They *wu* it and they *fu* it, they *ru* it and they *mo* it, and they use all sorts of dry-ing and heating drugs to attack it. They perform moxibustion on the middle of the belly, they burn the area below the navel, and they burn the *san li* point.[1] They *zheng* it and *yun* it, *tang* it and *kang* it."[2] *Wu, fu, ru*, and *mo* are shorthand for commonly used drug ingredients: *wu tou* and *fu zi*, types of monkshood or *Aconitum*; *ru xiang*, frankincense; and *mo yao*, myrrh. *Zheng, yun, tang*, and *kang* are all therapies that apply heat and drugs to the outside of the body in different ways. A foot qi sufferer, Zhang suggests, is willing to serially, indiscriminately experiment, ending up in such a state that "even if he ran into Bian Que or Hua Tuo," legendary doctors with almost magical skill, they would be unable to save him.[3] In reality, the therapies Zhang criticizes here as lacking a systematic therapeutic rationale seem relatively con-sistent. Monkshood has been used to expel cold and wind, frankin-cense and myrrh to promote circulation of blood and qi and alleviate pain. The externally applied heat therapies were also thought to help dispel cold influence near the surface of the body. If these were indeed popular responses to what people called foot qi, this further hints that what they were calling foot qi was not a vitamin deficiency disorder. Drugs such as the ones mentioned here would have no effect on a thiamine deficiency but might affect skin problems or arthritic pain.[4] But the foot qi that these popular therapies addressed is not recognized in either modern medicine or by Zhang Congzheng.

Foot qi, Zhang fumes, is not even a legitimate category of disease. The term does not appear in the *Yellow Emperor's Inner Canon*, the cardinal medical classic; it is nothing but a crude popular name that ignorant doctors use to label what are more rightly identified as manifestations of *bi*. Condemning the "erroneous and muddled theories of [his] contemporaries," Zhang writes,

> When people today edit formularies, whenever they see *bi* symptoms,[5] they just make them out to be foot qi and so treat them. Don't they know that there is no discussion of foot qi in the *Inner Canon*? . . . why is it that when they treat this, [my contemporaries] don't investigate the circulation tracts, don't discriminate the organ systems involved, don't distinguish between outer and inner, and just make it out to be cold-wet foot qi?[6]

The general outline of the situation—physician complains about rival methods for dealing with foot qi—resembles what we have already seen in the seventh century. The specifics, however—a doctor diagnosing "cold-wet foot qi," a patient trying a series of standard therapies—reflect changes that occurred in the intervening centuries. In particular, they reflect the way in which an ambitious government, promoting public health with unprecedented vigor, fostered a new genre that simplified and standardized medical knowledge.[7] The genre was the official drug formulary, compiled by government physicians to facilitate self-treatment and help relieve the burden of disease. The most influential of these formularies centered on the drugs available at the newly established imperial pharmacies. In the case of foot qi, the way the government formularies standardized knowledge later made some of it transferable to modernizing Western medicine in the late nineteenth century. The only feature of premodern concepts of foot qi that survived its modern transformation into beriberi is the idea that three main types of the disease can be distinguished: wet, dry, and fulminating (*chong xin*).

If one sees beriberi as the only correct meaning of foot qi, then the story presented here—of government officials simplifying and standardizing the definition of disease and creating types of a disease that are part of our modern understanding of beriberi today—looks like progress, an advance over the ambiguity of the texts we've examined so far. But viewing it that way allows one to miss a more interesting conclusion. The culture of government medicine in imperial China resembled the culture of modern biomedicine in that it was a highly bureaucratic system of healing that favored reduction and eschewed ambiguity. This characteristic shaped the way diseases were understood and treated in thirteenth-century China much as is it has shaped the way diseases are understood and treated today.

Drugs and Books: The Song Government's Medical Activism

The key period, the tenth through twelfth centuries, was a time of tremendous innovation in China, a period in which new staple crops, new educational opportunities, new technologies, and new forms of currency emerged. One reason for this dynamism was a shift that had begun centuries earlier. The preceding government, of the Tang empire, had eroded the power of the aristocratic families who had dominated the imperial political system for more than a millennium, bringing new blood into the government by making a competitive examination system central to official appointment. This change brought new ideas into the upper reaches of government, ideas that began to bear fruit in the subsequent Song period, when reformers rose to the highest official positions, promoted by emperors who shared their vision of a more expansive role for the state in guiding and supporting the people. Consequently, the Song state involved itself more actively in many areas—education, trade, lending, public welfare—than had any imperial government beforehand and than would any imperial government afterwards.[8]

Not surprisingly, this time was also characterized by intense factional strife. Conservatives opposed the reformers, and the group that one ruler warmly approved might be rejected by the next, so succession could bring dramatic purges and policy reversals. When the emperor Shenzong acceded to the throne in 1068, he appointed as chief councilor the reformer Wang Anshi, who promulgated a far-reaching series of changes known collectively as the New Policies. After Shenzong's death in 1085, Wang fell from power and was replaced by conservatives who eliminated or diminished many of the New Policies, but a few years later another power transition at the top brought the reformers back. Despite this lurching back and forth, however, on the whole the Northern Song was a time of active and expansive government. The northern half of the empire was conquered by invading Jurchens in 1127, at which point what remained of the regime fled south and regrouped, presiding over a territorially diminished empire for a century and a half before submitting to the Mongols in 1279.

The Song government involved itself in health care just as actively as it did in the economy and education. Some emperors took a personal interest in medicine, from the founding emperor Taizu (r. 960–976), who treated his younger brother, the future Emperor Taizong, with moxibustion and acupuncture; to Taizong (r. 976–997) himself, who collected medical formulas; to Huizong (r. 1101–1125), whose many intellectual pursuits included medicine.[9] But if their interest had been merely personal, it would have amounted to no more than Huizong's famous collection of garden rocks. They considered nurturing the health of their people a necessary element of governmental benevolence, incumbent on any ruler who wished to emulate the ancient Zhou dynasty, the model of virtuous rule.[10]

The Northern Song government promoted health among its subjects primarily by providing two things, drugs and books. Medical officials, in previous dynasties responsible for caring only for members of the court, now were regularly charged with distributing drugs to the people in the midst of epidemics.[11] More important, in 1076 the government established an imperial pharmacy with local branches that sold drug ingredients and prepared drug formulas all the time and not only during epidemic crises. As Asaf Goldschmidt has shown, the pharmacy began as a kind of market-regulating and moneymaking venture on the part of the government with, incidentally, a humanitarian purpose as well. It made standard drug formulas available year-round, at least to those within reach of a branch. The availability of fresh plant- and animal-derived drug ingredients had always been seasonal, but the personnel of official pharmacies systematically preserved such ingredients, stabilizing the supply somewhat. In addition, a patient could be fairly confident that the drugs acquired at an official pharmacy were not fake and that the price paid was fair, or at least controlled by government regulation. Outside of the pharmacy, the prices of drug ingredients tended to spike out of season or when demand suddenly increased; the pharmacy helped to counteract some of the typical price gouging.[12]

These significant advantages made the pharmacies popular enough to ensure their survival in spite of the brutal factionalism of Northern Song politics. The pharmacy system was one of the few policy changes enacted under Wang Anshi that outlasted his tenure. So popular was the system, in fact, that it survived even the conquest of the Northern Song by the Jurchens; the latter created their own version of the public pharmacies, whereas the remnants of the Northern Song regime who reestablished the government in the south built a new network of pharmacies there, ultimately expanding the system to seventy branches.[13]

In addition to providing drugs, the government also contributed to public health by producing medical books. Earlier regimes had undertaken similar projects, but Song emperors sponsored more of them than any of their predecessors, and they reached more readers and lasted longer than similar official works from earlier dynasties. Before the tenth century, such magisterial works had extremely limited distribution outside the palace, if they were distributed at all. They were tools of government primarily in the sense that they helped a dynasty advertise its legitimacy and power. The Tang government, for example, commissioned the disease encyclopedia we examined in the previous chapter, *Sources and Symptoms of All Disease*, as well as a massive volume of drug ingredients, the *Newly Revised Materia Medica* (*Xin xiu ben cao*). By collecting and producing such works, the reigning dynasty communicated that it had under its control not only the people and territory of the empire but also the intellectual heritage of Chinese civilization, including all that was known about the natural, historical, and social worlds.

The medical publishing projects of the Northern Song emperors went beyond legitimation, though; they affected doctors and a significant portion of the lay public, even in places far from Kaifeng, the capital. How? For one thing, their sheer number and volume eclipsed what earlier governments had produced. As TJ Hinrichs has tabulated, in the 350 years before the Song dynasty, Chinese governments commissioned only five medical texts, whereas, in the first two centuries of the Song, the government created thirty-four medical books, some revised and annotated classics and others completely new.[14] The very active Song Bureau for Revising Medical Texts was charged with revising, annotating, and reissuing rare but important books in the imperial library. Many of the books it produced—such as the *Yellow Emperor's Inner Canon* or the *A-B Classic* (*Jia yi jing*)—had been passed on in variant versions over the centuries through master–disciple lineages. The Bureau for Revising Medical Texts standardized the form and content of these books and broadened their use beyond the scattered lineages of initiated doctors. Many of the versions of early medical texts that have been passed down to modern times achieved their standard form during the Song period. Although we do not know how much money or personnel Song emperors allotted to the Bureau for Revising Medical Texts, judging from the number of major works it produced in the second half of the eleventh century, it must have been considerable.

In addition, the government's biggest medical projects, the official formularies, had a practical purpose quite apart from the symbolic prestige that accrued to collecting and displaying natural knowledge. Chapters One and Two have introduced the genre of formularies, practical compendia of drugs and techniques associated with particular sets of symptoms. The examples we have seen there, Ge Hong's *Emergency Formulas to Keep up Your Sleeve* and Sun Simiao's *Formulas Worth a Thousand in Gold*, were created by eminent individuals as a humanitarian act. In the Song period, the formularies compiled by the government made the biggest impact.

The Emperor Taizong, who reportedly collected more than a thousand medical formulas himself, enthusiastically promoted the creation of such compendia. He issued an edict offering a reward to those who submitted private medical books to the court, either as a donation or to be copied and returned. The edict promised that medical texts amounting to 200 chapters or more would earn the donor promotion and remuneration if he were an official, and official appointment if he were not.[15] Taizong then ordered medical officials in the Hanlin Academy to compile two formularies based on the emperor's own collection, the texts of the imperial library, and the books that his subjects had submitted in response to the edict. The first of these projects to reach completion, an enormous thousand-chapter work completed in 986, is no longer extant despite its size. The second formulary, a more modest hundred-chapter compendium compiled in 992, survives intact today. This was the *Imperial Grace Formulary of the Great Peace and Prosperous State Era* (*Tai ping sheng hui fang*, hereafter *Imperial Grace Formulary*). The emperor seems to have intended this formulary to be used, and not just to bolster government prestige; once it was finished he had it copied and the copies transported to the headquarters of provincial officials. But knowing how precious books were, provincial officials tended to take preservation, not dissemination, as their main task. They kept the *Imperial Grace Formulary*, once copied, locked up to protect it from wind and weather—and commoners.[16]

About a hundred years later, however, medical officials working under the direction of Emperor Huizong (r. 1101–1125) published a third imperial formulary, and this one became very popular in the twelfth and thirteenth centuries and influenced medical literature long afterward. This was the *Pharmacy Formulary of the Great Peace and Prosperous State Era* (*Tai ping hui min he ji ju fang*, hereafter *Pharmacy Formulary*), first printed in 1110.[17] The *Pharmacy Formulary* was more useful to individuals as a manual for self-treatment than previous official formularies had been. First of all, it is much simpler than its precursors, which had discussed pulse types and medical theory; the *Pharmacy Formulary* leaves out such specialized knowledge. It also reduces the number of formulas suggested for each disease to a convenient small set. For foot qi, for example, where the eighth-century *Arcane Essentials of the Imperial Library* had described sixty-four different formulas, and the tenth-century *Imperial Grace Formulary* seventy-three, the *Pharmacy Formulary* pared down the relevant treatments to only twenty-one.

More significantly, the *Pharmacy Formulary* was based on an inventory of the new state-run pharmacies, which meant that the potions, powders, pills, and ointments that it recommended were available at these institutions. So if the *Pharmacy Formulary* recommended Gold Sprouts Wine, Banksia Rose Pills, Noble Dendrobium Powder, or Rhinoceros Horn Decoction,[18] and one lived within reach of a state pharmacy, one could buy the drug there, already compounded. This made the *Pharmacy Formulary* more immediately useful than any previous formulary had been and contributed to its enormous success. Southern Song emperors commissioned the equivalent of second, third, and fourth editions as a demonstration of their benevolence. The book was so influential that some historians of Chinese medicine write about the twelfth and thirteenth centuries as the era of "*Pharmacy Formulary* medicine."[19]

If its simplified content and its connection with the pharmacies made the formulary broadly useful, woodblock printing extended its reach. Before the tenth century, virtually all books in China had been manuscripts, texts handwritten on paper, silk, or—in ancient times— slats of wood or bamboo. By the eighth century AD, a form of printing had emerged: woodblock, different from the movable type that would emerge many centuries later in Europe. To produce a woodblock print, a scribe first wrote out a page of text by hand on paper. The page was then affixed to a specially prepared block of wood, and carvers whittled away the wood around the characters, leaving a panel of raised text. Printers made copies by inking the carved block and pressing paper against it. Depending on the quality of the wood, a set of blocks could produce anywhere from 6,000 to 40,000 prints before it became blurry and unusable.[20]

In its first century or so, woodblock printing had mostly been used by individuals and monasteries to reproduce religious texts. Reproducing the word of the Buddha was a merit-earning act that could help improve one's own lot or that of a relative after death, so the faithful and the fearful who had the means to do so had scriptures printed in abundance. By the early Song, however, the imperial government adopted the new technology to print secular texts. Editors working for the National Academy began to compare extant variants of books and to iron out the differences among them to print standard versions. They produced standard editions of dynastic histories and of the Confucian classics starting in the 980s.

Soon the official printing projects had diversified to incorporate works of natural and practical knowledge, including medical classics.[21] These were printed in large format using costly materials and were both unwieldy and expensive. Once the formal editions of official medical works were finished and entrusted to the imperial library, however, the Bureau for Revising Medical Texts proceeded to issue a set of relatively cheap small-character editions meant for wider circulation.[22] Private printers, a new industry, quickly followed up by cutting their own woodblock versions of official texts, often abridging them to make their content more accessible both intellectually and financially. By the twelfth and thirteenth centuries, phrases such as "abridged essentials" (*jie yao*) and "an outline of the essentials" (*lüe yao*) became common in the titles of medical works.

Like other official medical books, the *Pharmacy Formulary* spawned a host of modified and abridged editions. Among these, one of the most important was an offshoot called *Easy, Concise Formulas* (*Yi jian fang*) by Wang Shuo, a sometime alcohol commissioner in Lin'an prefecture (modern Hangzhou).[23] Written between 1190 and 1220, *Easy, Concise Formulas* was a one-chapter formulary that, true to its title, pared down the content of the *Pharmacy Formulary*—itself a streamlined version of earlier collections—even further. The number of recommended formulas for each condition diminished radically, in the case of foot qi dropping from the *Pharmacy Formulary*'s twenty-one to a mere six.[24] The entire book contains only thirty of the most commonly used formulas at the time, as compared with the 297 that the *Pharmacy Formulary* includes.

Easy, *Concise Formulas* ended up more widely used than the *Pharmacy Formulary* itself. The eminent poet Liu Chenweng wrote perhaps a half-century after the publication of Wang's book, "Since *Easy, Concise Formulas* started circulating, the four big formularies"—including the *Pharmacy Formulary*—"have all fallen out of use."[25] The book inspired another rash of books with variations on the same title, such as the *Expanded and Revised* Easy, Concise Formulas (*Zeng xiu yi jian fang*) and *Edited and Annotated Supplement to* Easy, Concise Formulas (*Jiao zheng zhu xu yi jian fang*). It also inspired several books criticizing Wang's work, a sure sign of its influence.[26]

The medical books that earlier Chinese governments had collected and commissioned had served to enhance the authority of the regime and to facilitate the treatment of a very limited number of elite patients. In the tenth through thirteenth centuries, however, the Song government undertook to disseminate medical texts to more of its subjects and make those texts easier to apply. Amplified by woodblock printing's publishing boom, these efforts put medical literature in more hands than ever before and equipped more laypeople with tools that facilitated self-treatment.

Accessible Empiricism: How *Pharmacy Formulary* Literature Informed Modern Medicine

The government formularies and their privately authored imitators did more than simply make the book knowledge of elite doctors available to a wider audience. The new formularies simplified and made explicit considerations involved in diagnosis and treatment that older texts had assumed required a doctor's discretion. They split diseases into a panoply of types that narrowed the range of possible diagnoses for a given patient regardless of the doctor's skill at reading the pulse. These texts present a checklist of symptoms as the central tool in therapeutic decision making and suggest standard drug formulas, available at the official pharmacies, as the main form of treatment. Their accessible empiricism rendered them comprehensible not only to laypeople in this period but also, eventually, to physicians in the nineteenth and twentieth centuries—as the case of foot qi attests.

The Song formularies divided diseases into types in a way that older texts had not. The *Pharmacy Formulary* discussion of foot qi, for example, distinguishes thirteen mutually exclusive types of the disease: there are wet, dry, and distressing-the-mind (*chong xin*) types of foot qi; yin and yang types; the rising qi type; one type assigned to each of the six "warps" (*jing*) of the body; and a Jiangdong-Lingnan miasmic type. Some of the distinctions among types of disease were straightforward, reflecting obvious symptoms or the geographical location of the sufferer. The difference between dry and wet foot qi, for example, was that "the dry one does not [involve] swelling; the wet one [involves] swelling and bloating."[27] Distressing-the-mind type was characterized by rapid and irregular heartbeat (the heart, not the brain, was considered the seat of consciousness and emotion). Jiangdong-Lingnan miasmic foot qi was by definition the type caused by the poisonous miasmas of the far southeast and hence could be contracted only there.[28] The rising qi type was identifiable by the location and sequence of obvious symptoms: pain in the feet moving up into the belly, followed by panting and heart palpitations.

Other types required a bit more detailed familiarity with medical concepts. Yin and yang qi, for example: the *Pharmacy Formulary* defines yin foot qi as the type located in the yin organ systems (known as *zang*), and yang foot qi as the type located in the yang organ systems (known as *fu*).[29] The *zang* organ systems—heart, liver, spleen, lung, and kidney[30]—were comparatively yin, the quality that traditional Chinese thought associates with latency, interiority, femininity, darkness, and the like. The *fu* systems—gall bladder, stomach, large intestine, small intestine, bladder, and triple *jiao*—were comparatively yang, associated with activity, exteriority, masculinity, and lightness.[31] Illness in the yin organ systems was relatively interior compared with illness in the yang organ systems and therefore more serious. The six "warps" (*jing*) were also a technical concept; the term originated in weaving, in which warp and weft threads together make up the cloth. In the body, the equivalent of the warp thread was the circulatory tract (sometimes called meridian or channel) along which qi was presumed to flow, producing the fabric of tissue and bone. The *Pharmacy Formulary* does, in other words, presume some degree of familiarity with the concepts of classical medicine—or at least presumes that its audience is mixed and will include classical practitioners.

Most of the information that the Song formularists drew on to create their types had been present in the seventh-century texts we have already examined, Chao Yuanfang's *Sources and Symptoms of All Disease* and Sun Simiao's *Formulas Worth a Thousand in Gold.* But the older texts had deployed that information in a way that required the judgment of the seasoned practitioner, whereas the new types made a physician's expertise more dispensable. For example, Sun Simiao had observed that foot qi patients sometimes experienced foot swelling and sometimes did not, but he emphasized that this was why the diagnosis should be left to a physician who would read the pulse and plumb the deeper pattern before making a judgment. A superficial symptom such as foot swelling would not lead the competent physician astray as it might a layperson. In the *Imperial Grace Formulary,* however, foot swelling becomes the signal symptom a reader can use to distinguish wet foot qi from dry. Likewise, the symptoms associated with rising foot qi are familiar from earlier books, but in earlier literature they had been a reason to take the disease seriously in its early stages, not a way to identify a type of foot qi and the appropriate drugs for it. In the fourth century, Ge Hong had warned, "If you don't treat [foot qi] immediately, [the qi] will turn and head upward, entering the belly, and then [the patient] will breathe heavily, and it will kill the person."[32] By contrast, in the Song formularies, these symptoms are not the fatal culmination of a disease inadequately treated but the signature of one particular type, for which drug formulas are available to try. The pattern is clear: Sun Simiao wrote that foot qi was not confined to a single region, so the Song formularists make the foot qi of the south into a distinct type. Sun Simiao wrote that women might be more susceptible to the disease after childbirth, so female foot qi and postchildbirth foot qi become types discussed in the burgeoning new literature on *fuke*, women's medicine.[33] The new Song formularies embrace the notion that foot qi has multiple manifestations but suggest that one need not understand the complex disorder that underlies them all. Treating the particular set of symptoms identified will suffice.

The *Pharmacy Formulary* genre prioritizes signals for the reader. It creates a dichotomous key for identifying disease entities, similar to what an amateur naturalist might use to identify a species of tree today. Just as knowing whether the leaves on a tree are lobed or nonlobed will send the naturalist to a subsection containing only one kind of tree, from which point further distinctions narrow the possibilities correspondingly, observing that the lower legs are swollen would send the would-be healer to the wet foot qi section of the formulary. From there, checking off other, less obvious symptoms allows the reader to choose one of fifteen subtypes. In this way, the reader can diagnose the condition without taking into consideration the complicated factors that a physician was supposed to weigh alongside the outward symptoms—the patient's constitution and habits, the progression of the illness, the season and climate, and the character of the pulse.

Of course, having a name to put to a sick person's condition is of little use if one does not also have a strategy for treating it. The government formularies accordingly supply the strategy. The *Pharmacy Formulary* and the *Easy, Concise Formulas* establish a clear, straightforward relationship between standard types and treatments. The *Pharmacy Formulary* groups disease into ten broad divisions, including "various wind disorders," "cold damage disorders," "all *qi* disorders," "phlegm disorders," and others. To find an appropriate treatment, one can begin from the general category of disease and skim the descriptions of the drugs included in that category. Each drug formula begins with a brief description of the symptoms and diseases it can treat effectively and then lists the ingredients used in the formula, followed by instructions—unnecessary if one were buying the compound from a state pharmacy—on how to prepare and administer the compound. If the general category of disease does not satisfactorily describe the patient's symptoms, one can move on to the types and subtypes of the disease. In the example given earlier, each of the fifteen subtypes of wet foot qi is associated with a single recommended drug formula.

Earlier texts had also connected syndromes to drug treatments. That was, after all, the raison d'être of the formulary genre and of many early medical texts. But the earlier texts had connected them to pulse types, as we have seen in Chao Yuanfang's *Sources and Symptoms of All Disease*: if the pulse were floating, one would use a different drug formula than if it were sinking, regardless of whether the external signs were otherwise identical.[34] Consider the contrast with the "Comprehensive Discussion of Guidelines" appended by Xu Hong to the *Imperial Grace Formulary* in 1208. The "Guidelines" discuss how to create prescriptions, how to combine and administer drugs, and how to recognize the symptoms of different types of disease. They then specify which formulas each type calls for—all described in the main text of the formulary. For foot qi, the "Guidelines" say:

> For the wet and swelling one, you can give Astragalus Root Building-the-Center Decoction or Lesser Life-Extending Decoction. For the wind and wet one, you can use Atractylodes Aconite Decoction. For the hot and thirst-inducing one, you can give Purple Snow. For the one associated with a distressed mind and depression, you can use Triple Harmony Powder or Hemp Seed Pills or Qi-lowering Decoction. For the one that involves a pain like a lower back injury, you can use Big Black Agar Wood Decoction.[35]

Here, the recommended formulas are associated with superficial symptoms that any layperson, including the patient him- or herself, can ascertain, rather than the pulse that only an experienced physician can read. For literate laypeople, the essays that Xu Hong appended made the formulary easy to use without the help of a doctor; one could locate the most salient symptom and then decide, based on the finer distinctions, which formula to try, skipping back to the main text to read about what the drug contained and how to compound it if necessary.

Classically educated doctors responded to the *Pharmacy Formulary* and its knockoffs with ambivalence or even hostility.[36] One might have expected Song physicians to discuss the pharmacy and its accompanying formulary as significant new resources, but in fact this important institution—amply mentioned in nonmedical texts—is virtually absent from their writings. Goldschmidt suggests that the *Pharmacy Formulary* did affect literati physicians' practice and outlook, but they saw the effect as mostly negative: it increased competition in the medical marketplace by empowering less educated healers to prescribe standard remedies. That is why they hardly ever brought it up, and they defended their own expertise by emphasizing their knowledge of the classics.[37] Thus Zhang Congzheng's complaint that opened this chapter: the *Pharmacy Formulary* and its imitators had enabled his contemporaries to simplify complicated experiences into simple disease varieties such as "cold wet foot qi," and treat them with standard remedies. They had begun to ignore the pulse, season, patient's constitution, or any of the myriad other variables that could render rote treatments ineffective or even lethal.[38]

Nevertheless, despite later Chinese physicians' aspersions on this period as one that contributed little to medical theory and even degraded medical practice, the accessible empiricism of these texts gave them a lasting legacy. In the case of foot qi, the disease types that Song formularies created constitute some of the only features of the classical disease that survived its transformation into biomedicine's beriberi many hundreds of years later. Beriberi today, like the foot qi in Song formularies, comes in wet and dry varieties distinguished by the symptom of lower leg swelling, as well as a form called fulminating beriberi, based on the *chong xin* type discussed in the Song formularies. Dry beriberi's hallmark, modern biomedical textbooks say, is damage and disruption to the nervous system, marked by the sharp and aching pain its sufferers experience as the nerves deteriorate. It is thought to be caused by a diet short of both calories and thiamine. Wet beriberi's symptoms center on the cardiovascular system and include high blood pressure, edema, and chest pain. These symptoms are thought to be caused by a diet that provides sufficient calories but lacks thiamine. As for "fulminant cardiovascular beriberi," biomedical textbooks are ambivalent about whether it is a separate type. It manifests just as Chao Yuanfang described the acute phase of foot qi back in 610—producing symptoms from anxiety and rapid heartbeat to bulging neck veins and blue extremities and threatening death if treatment is administered inappropriately or too slowly. But it is unclear whether fulminant beriberi has a different cause, as wet and dry beriberi are presumed to, or is simply the end stage of either wet or dry beriberi.

The preservation of these types does not mean that Song dynasty foot qi and modern beriberi are biologically the same disease. Some Song foot qi may well have been beriberi. But it is impossible to make a positive diagnosis based on the simple assertion that "the dry one does not [involve] swelling; the wet one [involves] swelling and bloating."[39] This description could apply to many diseases other than beriberi, including diabetes, heart disease, or gout. What it does show is something about how *Pharmacy Formulary* medicine resembles modern biomedicine.

In biomedicine today, types of disease are common and are reflected in the disease codes of the International Classification of Diseases (ICD) system. The system distinguishes type I from type II diabetes, for example (ICD-9 codes 250.01 and 250.00, respectively), defining one as the kind caused by the body's failure to produce insulin, generally first appearing in childhood, and the other as the kind caused by too little insulin or the body's failure to respond to insulin, generally first appearing in adults. The types are recognized as related but distinct. Types proliferate in modern biomedicine, each edition of the ICD containing more codes than the previous one, so that what began as a list of a few hundred disease classifications in 1898 had grown to thousands of distinctions by the time the ICD-10 was completed in 1992.[40] This expansion reflects a bureaucratic imperative for ever-greater precision, as the codes serve to connect the increasingly complex empire of health care providers with the increasingly complex empire of insurers. In Song China the bureaucratic imperative was of a different scale, but types of disease proliferated in a similar manner. The group of officials tasked with producing the *Pharmacy Formulary*, in fact, faced a similar challenge to the one that the disease-classification committee of the International Statistics Conference did when charged with creating the first version of the ICD in the 1890s: how to make disease types that were uniformly recognizable.

Both *Pharmacy Formulary* medicine and modern biomedicine are characterized by a reductionist impulse, an attempt to make a complex phenomenon universally legible by breaking it down into constituent parts or types. Both also respond to a bureaucratic imperative to make diagnosis simpler and more objective, so that (in the case of the Song formularies) patients can directly benefit from the government's benevolence or (in the case of modern beriberi) classes of medical students can grasp the appropriate treatment rationale quickly, and health care providers can communicate precisely with insurers. Earlier texts such as the *Formulas Worth a Thousand in Gold* had offered a thickly layered description of foot qi, its manifestations, and its remedies, assuming that the practitioner's accumulated experience and education would enable him to identify the most relevant data in any given case. But this kind of knowledge is not well suited to a standardized text for a lay autodidact or for first-year medical students trying to absorb and retain information about disease symptoms for class exams. A great deal of personal tutelage is needed to order and activate the information in the reader's mind. Not surprisingly, then, this sort of content did not survive foot qi's translation into Song formulary literature or into modern medicine. Nor, for that matter, did the Song types that rely on classical medical theory, such as yin and yang foot qi and foot qi associated with the six warps. They have been discarded, as has Lingnan-Jiangdong foot qi, because environment is considered irrelevant to beriberi.

The twelfth century marks a high point of government medical activism. After that, the imperial government's medical initiatives diminished in scope and number, leaving public health in late imperial China in the hands of private philanthropists.[41] After the final collapse of the Song government in 1279, the imperial pharmacy system dwindled and disappeared, and no emperor again commissioned medical officials to revise and reissue the pharmacy formulary. The division of foot qi into types, however, carried over into late imperial China, as wet and dry, *chong xin*, yin and yang, and other types persisted in later books. In addition, thirteenth-century authors drew on the Song formulary precedent to delineate a new type of foot qi distinguished by its cause: internal foot qi brought on by a faulty diet. This form of foot qi would become the object of a great deal of attention and debate by the sixteenth century, reflecting the social and economic changes that were upending traditional hierarchies in late Ming China. That change is the subject of the next chapters.

CHAPTER FOUR

The Northerner's Dietary Disorder

In its earliest incarnation, as we have seen in Chapter One, foot qi was considered peculiar to the south, one of the many ailments that menaced migrants in the lush landscape beyond the Yangzi River. But before long it became clear that one could develop foot qi even in the familiar and civilized environment of the north. This long puzzled physicians. Between the fourth and thirteenth centuries, they made a number of attempts to explain it, generally by asserting that the environmental qi that caused the disease was spreading to new areas. Sun Simiao asserted in the seventh century that qi in different regions, formerly more distinct, had homogenized as Tang emperors consolidated their rule. A few centuries later, the physicians whom the second Song emperor commissioned to write the *Imperial Grace Formulary* wrote, "Wind poison moves everywhere under heaven. It is not just in Jiangdong and Lingnan."[1]

As time went on, though, explanations for the conundrum of foot qi in the north began to point toward an entirely new theory of causation, one connected not to environmental qi but to diet. In the eleventh century, the physician Dong Ji, author of *Comprehensive Essentials for Treating Foot Qi* (*Jiao qi zhi fa zong yao*), reported that he'd contracted foot qi himself in the snows of what is now western Shandong province, well to the north of the region traditionally implicated. Like Sun, he thought political consolidation had had epidemiological consequences—but, rather than an abstract homogenization of environmental qi, he pointed to more concrete effects: since the Song emperors had reunified China in AD 960, he wrote, "There is no difference in foodstuffs between north and south, and roads are not limited by being long and remote." That meant that more northerners were traveling south, more southerners traveling north, and people in one region were eating foods better suited to people from another region, with the result that, in recent years, many "in the interior regions," formerly unaffected, had contracted foot qi.[2]

By the thirteenth century, the hint that human habits, not environmental conditions, caused some cases of foot qi developed into a fully articulated theory that distinguished a distinctive northern type of disease. Li Gao (aka Li Dongyuan, 1180–1251), one of the most prominent scholar-physicians during a time noted for innovation in Chinese medicine, posited that northerners contracted foot qi by eating and drinking too much. Li's creation of northern foot qi reflected how the political, economic, and cultural division of the Han Chinese population starting in the tenth century had produced distinctive northern and southern Chinese identities. North and south had become more medically meaningful than ever before, and hints in early medical classics that northerners' bodies and diseases differed from southerners' began to be elaborated in more concrete ways.

Scholars who have examined the history of foot qi have generally ignored or downplayed the developments in this chapter and the next, treating the dietary foot qi that thirteenth- through nineteenth-century Chinese sources describe as irrelevant to the disease's true history because records of foot qi in this period insufficiently evoke beriberi.[3] The twentieth-century scholar Chen Bangxian, for example, complained that twelfth-century foot qi discussions "muddled" together diverse conditions such as "edema, foot pain, and beriberi," and that later medical books applied the name foot qi to what was clearly arthritis.[4] In contrast, refusing to naturalize the modern translation of foot qi as its proper meaning through all of time allows us to take late imperial foot qi seriously and to explore the social and intellectual contexts in which novel theories of disease flourished in China without arrogantly disparaging those theories as incorrect.

Northern Stomachs and Spleens:
A New Pathway for Dangerous Qi

Li Gao was one of the most eminent physicians of the thirteenth century, recognized generations after his death as one of the "four great doctors" of the twelfth through fourteenth centuries. The "four greats" advanced new approaches to disease that reinvigorated medical doctrine in the face of the *Pharmacy Formulary*–dominated medicine whose development the previous chapter outlined.[5] When it came to foot qi, Li accepted the theory of causation that had been passed down in nearly a millennium's worth of medical literature—that the disease was generally caused by invasive qi steaming up from the ground into the feet and lower legs. This, he wrote, clearly explained its occurrence in the south. But he thought people in the north were unlikely to contract a disease through contact with damp earth. In the arid north, the poisonous qi characteristic of the "low and wet terrain in the south where fog and mist collect" was rare.[6] Moreover, northerners' bodies were different, less permeable, than those of southerners. According to a contemporaneous source preserved in a later compilation, southerners were practically built to absorb illness-causing qi: "The people [in the south] have loose pores, and their yang qi is not able to block off the outside of their bodies [that is, keep pernicious qi from entering], so when they tread on [the low, wet terrain of the south], the cold and wet qi attack them, and the disease rises from below."[7] Northerners, Li contended, had tighter pores and therefore were less vulnerable to invasive qi. And yet it was common knowledge that they too suffered from foot qi. Li articulates this conundrum in the form of an unnamed observer's objection: "Someone asks a difficult question: today in the north, the land is high and cold, and the people's pores are fine (*zhi mi*). Yet still many of them have this disease. Is this because they contract the wet qi of the earth?"[8]

Li's reply: no. Northerners get foot qi because they "regularly consume koumiss, and drink without moderation."[9] It is their habits, not their constitution or their environment, that bring about their suffering. This represents a significant change in the perception of the disease as well as in the perception of the relationship between diet and illness.

Considering the political circumstances prevailing in his time, and the originality of his thought, it is no surprise either that Li Gao took special notice of a north–south difference in a disease or that he came up with a novel explanation for that difference. Li lived in an area of north China that is in today's Hebei province, not far from Beijing, a setting in which differences between the people of northern and southern China were growing more apparent and more meaningful than they had been before. Chinese literati had long thought of north and south as distinct parts of the empire, but the meaning of that division changed greatly as political and social boundaries shifted. As we have seen in Chapter One, in the fourth century when the first written records of foot qi emerged, most of the Chinese population was still located in the north China plain surrounding the Yellow River. A long migration south had already begun, however, and although northerners long continued to view the south with anxiety and disapprobation, by the eleventh century travel between north and south had become increasingly easy and frequent. The Song state (960–1279) effectively governed Fujian, Guangxi, and other far-south regions for the first time. Northern officials served in the south and vice versa. In the flourishing economy of the tenth and eleventh centuries, empirewide markets distributed the goods and commodities of all regions.

This peaceable picture changed significantly in the twelfth and thirteenth centuries. A series of non-Chinese regimes emerged from the Manchurian forests and the Mongolian steppe on the frontiers of the Chinese empire, and they quickly expanded to conquer territory in the northern part of the Song state.[10] The Liao dynasty (AD 916–1125) was headed by a family of Khitan nomads who maintained one type of government for the sedentary Chinese and another for the nomads to the north. The rulers of the Jin dynasty, a family of Jurchen tribesmen from Manchuria (AD 1115–1234), eventually conquered the Liao and extended their rule in Li Gao's north China. It was a period in which the Chinese empire found itself, as the historian Morris Rossabi has put it, "among equals."[11]

Once the Jin conquered the north in the early twelfth century, people who lived north of the Huai River and people who lived south of it inhabited two different empires, one ruled by Chinese and the other by Jurchen. Goods and people no longer passed freely between these areas. By Li Gao's time, northern and southern China had been separated for over a hundred years—or more than 300, for those living farther north in former Liao dynasty territory. Han Chinese such as Li had been subjects of non-Chinese northerners all their lives, as had their parents and grandparents. Region and ethnicity-based caste had become part of their everyday experience. Differences between Chinese and non-Chinese, and between northern and southern Chinese, therefore figured prominently in the way such people understood the world, and the definition of disease was one manifestation of that worldview. Thus, regional divisions gained new prominence in twelfth-century medicine.

Region had, to be sure, factored into earlier medical theory and practice, as we have seen in Chapter One. As early as the *Yellow Emperor's Inner Canon* medical writers had asserted that constitutions, habits, illnesses, and appropriate therapies varied from region to region. Earlier literature had discussed both five-region divisions (north, south, east, west, center) and the north–south division, the former more important as part of an abstract universal theory and the latter mattering more in practice. In Li Gao's time, medical writers continued to discuss both models; just as in earlier literature, five regions fulfilled a theoretical imperative whereas north–south fulfilled a practical one. In this period the unifying theory of which five regions formed a part was the *wu yun liu qi* system, sometimes translated "phase energetics." This was a means of predicting epidemics according to year and season by combining the five phases with the ten celestial stems, and the six types of climatic qi with the twelve earthly branches. In other words, it represented the same kind of attempt to regularize the infinite variety of the natural world that the original five-phase system of the *Inner Canon* did, but it was more numerologically complex.[12] It had begun to appear in the Song and by the eleventh century was extremely popular among medical writers, who described its elaborate calculations and correspondences with verve. Enterprising authors inserted new essays on phase energetics into the *Yellow Emperor's Inner Canon*, where most modern versions of the classic retain them today. The influence of phase energetics pervades the official *Medical*

Encyclopedia: A Sagely Benefaction (*Sheng ji zong lu*) compiled in
1111–1117; the very first chapter is an essay on the topic. A common
saying among doctors around this time was "If you don't study phase
energetics, what help can you provide even if you have examined every
formulary?"[13] Phase energetics encouraged Jin and Yuan dynasty doctors to write about geography as an idealized, five-part whole.

Still, as in the earlier period, for many medical writers the north–
south division mattered more. For example, in his pediatric treatise
Oral Comments on Saving Children's Lives (*Huo you kou yi*, 1332), author Zeng Shirong mentions both regional patterns but clearly views
the north–south division as the one of primary importance. He dutifully recites the association between different foods and the cardinal
directions: "Northern fruits are mostly cooling; southern fruits are
mostly heating; eastern fruits are mostly sour; and western fruits are
mostly astringent." But he then goes on to explain, with a good deal
more fervor, how southerners and northerners misunderstand the
food of the other region: "Southerners cannot eat northern things.
They take flour staples to be a fine food, and jujubes (Chinese dates)
to be a vegetable. And how can northerners eat southern things, when
they take fish to be a green vegetable, and toads to be rice?"[14]

The tension apparent in the previous discussion—between fidelity to five-phase correspondence theory and empirical observation
of north–south difference—is as visible in the foot qi literature as in
the rest of the medical corpus. Because foot qi originally appeared in
formularies, the most practical of medical genres, it is not surprising
that its original geographical association was specific and concrete and
had nothing to do with five-phase theory. Ge Hong matter-of-factly
linked it to the region just south of the Yangzi River. Many authors
in subsequent centuries reiterated Ge's geographical parameters, but
a few noted that the same condition seemed to exist outside of the
south. It was Li Gao, however, who first combined the geographical
observations of the early foot qi literature with the theory of regional
constitutions in the *Yellow Emperor's Inner Canon*. As his authority on
"the sources from which one contracts northern foot qi," Li cites the
Inner Canon. But the specific characteristics that he associates with

northern and southern people, and northern and southern foot qi, do not tally with the *Inner Canon's* discussion.

The passages in the *Inner Canon* discussion directly relevant to the north–south distinction read as follows:

In the north is the area where heaven and earth close up and store. The land is high, people live in the hills, and the wind and cold are freezing. The people there enjoy wild places and eat dairy foods. The cold that they [thus] store up fills them up with diseases. To treat such diseases it is appropriate to use moxibustion, so moxibustion comes from the north.

In the south is the place where heaven and earth nourish one another and yang flourishes. The land there is low and the environment fragile; it is a place where fog and mist collect. The people there love sour [foods] and eat fermented things. They all have fine pores [*zhi li*] and red faces, and their illnesses are *luan* [twitching, convulsions] and *bi* [a deep and persistent achiness]. To treat such diseases it is appropriate to needle slightly, so the nine needles come from the south.[15]

Li's southerners have loose pores, but the southerners in the *Inner Canon* have fine spaces in the skin. In fact, the *Inner Canon* uses the same adjective to describe southerners' pores that Li uses to describe northerners': *zhi*, fine or closely spaced. His northerners do eat dairy foods and live in cold hills, like the northerners in the *Inner Canon*, but according to the *Inner Canon* it should be westerners, not northerners, who are susceptible only to internally caused diseases. Westerners do not exist in Li's rubric, however, which takes into consideration not five regions but two. Region clearly mattered to Li Gao, but he uses the *Inner Canon's* discussion of region merely to give the appearance of according with classical theory. In reality, three of its five regions are superfluous to his observations about regional forms of foot qi, and the constitutions and symptoms he writes about differ markedly from those described in the venerable classic.

These examples from Li's and Zeng's books, in which they dutifully recite characteristics associated with the classical five regions but describe north–south differences more enthusiatically, are typical of literature in this period. Physicians' theories—particularly phase energetics—called for a balance among five units, but the north–south division was more germane to their practice and lived experience. The real world, reflecting the conquest of the north by non-Chinese peoples and the political and economic rise of the south, was cleft in two, not five. The political context helps explain why the old puzzle about foot qi—if qi peculiar to the south caused it, how did people in the north get it?—had new prominence and why Li was inclined to explain it as a difference between two fundamentally distinct kinds of people.

Li's explanation derives also from the distinctive theories about illness that he had cultivated throughout his career. In his most influential work, the *Treatise on the Spleen and Stomach* (*Pi wei lun*), Li elevated the spleen and stomach organ systems to central importance in keeping the body healthy. The spleen and stomach were thought to be responsible for refining the qi of food and drink by cooking it, the first step in transforming it into the qi of the body. These organ systems thus contributed to the orderly circulation of energies and substances that kept a body vital. For that reason, damage to the spleen and stomach was particularly detrimental: it could slow down or obstruct the whole system, throwing it into chaos. The result could be "intense generalized fever, headache . . . dizziness, heavy limbs, debilitated limbs, fatigue, and somnolence."[16] From Li's perspective, damage to spleen and stomach was generally self-inflicted, brought on by "dietary irregularity and lack of moderation in [eating] cold and hot [foods]." Spleen and stomach "insufficiency" could also cause problems, and these usually resulted from too little yang qi and too much yin qi in the body.[17] He downplayed invasive external qi, arguing that if the body's internal transformations and circulation were proceeding smoothly, external qi could do no harm.

Li Gao brought his theories about spleen, stomach, food, and drink to bear on the question of northern foot qi, which he addressed in a slim volume called *Medical Theory Made Clear* (*Yi xue fa ming*). He wrote the book near the end of his life, and a disciple edited and published it after his death.[18] By the time a second disciple converted it into a woodblock print in 1279, thereby increasing the likelihood that what was left of the manuscript would survive, most of its original content had already disappeared.[19] As is often the case, however, parts of the lost sections were preserved in later works. *Excellent, Remarkably Effective Formulas* (*Qi xiao liang fang*, hereafter *Excellent Formulas*), a Ming government–sponsored formulary completed in 1471, is the best source of such fragments, and the quotations from *Medical Theory Made Clear* preserved there help us understand Li's new form of foot qi a little better.

Medical Theory Made Clear suggested that the foot qi caused by an invasion of deviant qi from the outside—the familiar etiology for the previous 500 years—was only one of two major types. The other "materializes from the inside." In particular, eating and drinking too much could induce the disease, if a person were unfortunate enough to have a weak stomach system:

> [Normally,] when people's food and drink enters their stomachs, stomach qi rises like a vapor. The qi and sapors [of the food and drink] are dispersed into the circulation tracts, where they are transformed into the yin and yang qi of the body. [But] if the body's primordial [*yuan*] qi[20] is insufficient, if the stomach system is weak at the root, and one increases [the amount] one eats and drinks, then the spleen and stomach systems will be injured. The qi and sapors [of food and drink] will not be able to disperse and circulate freely.[21]

If they were not adequately robust to begin with, the spleen and stomach systems—which normally received, digested, and dispersed the qi of food and drink—would not be able to handle much material at one time. A backlog in the stomach would hamper the spleen, which waited to receive the incoming qi for further refining. As the system slowed and weakened, substances that normally "disperse[d] and circulate[d] freely" would begin to collect in the lower extremities. The feet would swell, the skin grow taut, and the calves and feet painful. Voilà: a case of foot qi.

Li's theory was by any measure a radical departure from earlier ideas about foot qi and from earlier ideas about the relationship between diet and disease too. Ge Hong's fourth-century account, examined in Chapter One, mentions nothing about diet. True, some of the remedies he proposes—such as fermented soybeans steeped in wine—sound as much like food as like medicine. That is typical of classical medicine, however, and does not indicate that Ge believed foot qi had a special relationship with diet. In the seventh century, Sun Simiao recommended and prohibited specific foods for foot qi: onions, fermented soybeans, chives, ginger, and orange peel among the recommendations, and meat, wine, and butter among the prohibitions.[22] As with Ge Hong's recommendations, however, one cannot conclude that Sun thought of foot qi as a diet-induced disease. He does not say that eating the prohibited foods causes foot qi or that failing to eat the recommended foods does. Instead, the list is a guide to improving one's prospects of recovery after having contracted the disease. Moreover, it was common for medical authors to proscribe heavy and oily foods (meats, butter) and wine for patients with all sorts of illnesses, not just foot qi.

Around the same time as Sun was writing his book, Su Jing warned foot qi sufferers against eating "things difficult to digest" and also offered them advice about when to eat: "[When a person] suffers foot qi, it is best if in the morning he eats whatever he likes until he is full, in the afternoon a little, and late in the day no more. If he is hungry he can eat soybean paste or porridge."[23] Like Sun's diet-related injunctions, Su's instructions do not suggest that dietary habits have brought about the disease. In sum, what these early passages describe is a disease that is neither more nor less related to diet than most others. Poor diet, like sexual profligacy and uncontrolled emotions, predisposed people to any number of syndromes and also hindered recovery. But Li Gao's "internal injury" theory goes much further, proposing that diet is not just important in convalescence but might by itself cause this particular disease.

Different as it is from previous theories, Li's idea retains a connection with them: its attention to moisture. Li saw overeating as the root of many different kinds of ailments, but what distinguished foot qi from other spleen- and stomach-damage disorders was what *kinds* of things the sufferer consumed excessively. Substances that, in his words, "have the form and properties of water" were especially problematic; popular drinks like koumiss (fermented mare's milk) and wine fit into this category.[24] Imbibing too much of them could lead to the characteristic lower leg and foot symptoms of foot qi—the swelling and the pain. The earlier sources had also warned of the danger of water-like substances, describing foot qi as something one caught in moist places, by being too long in contact with damp earth, the vapors of which could rise into the feet. Most had agreed that the causative qi was wind, but some had described it, instead, as wet qi or wind-and-wet. All agreed that moisture was involved. Although he implicitly rejected the old idea that wind qi migrating around the empire had extended foot qi's reach, Li embraced the equally old idea that wet qi was involved. But wet qi did not only enter the body through the feet and through the spaces in the skin, according to Li; sometimes it entered through the mouth in the form of drink.

Li Gao's belief that northerners and southerners were built differently and lived differently thus allowed him to propose a novel theory of causation without rejecting the older theory outright. This perspective proved enormously influential through late imperial China, when regional styles of therapy flourished. The styles of therapy associated with the "four great doctors" came to be perceived as appropriate for people from one region but not for people from the other. One of the "four greats," Zhang Congzheng, whom we met in the previous chapter, espoused attacking and expelling pernicious qi as the first step of therapy. Only then could the patient begin to recover. Another, Zhu Zhenheng, took a different tack, preferring to replenish the patient's own qi with tonics enabling her body to cast out the illness-causing qi as a matter of course, without resorting to harsh purgatives. Because Zhang Congzheng, like Li Gao, lived in the north in territory under Jin dynasty rule, his "attacking and purging school" (*gong xia pai*) came to be considered a kind of northern therapy, whereas Zhu's "nourishing yin qi school" (*yang yin pai* or *zi yin pai*) became known as a southern therapy. Although the approach to treatment elucidated in their work is subtler and more complicated than simply purging versus replenishing, in effect these authors were made into the standard-bearers for contrasting regional orientations to treatment.

The impulse to create a special northern therapy for the northern syndrome appeared as early as internal foot qi itself. Li Gao believed that this therapy "should naturally be different from [that for] the southern disease,"²⁵ but the extant scraps of his book tell us no more than that. None of its six surviving formulas indicates that they are specifically for northern or for southern foot qi. A century and a half later, the *Universal Aid Formulary* asserted that there was still no standard remedy for northern foot qi. According to the formulary's editors,

> The Classic says: When the foot and calf swell, this is called water; [disorder in the] Mature Yin tract brings about swelling in the instep. This only refers to the kind [of foot qi] that enters from the outside. Its methods of treatment have been completely described in the formularies by earlier people. As for the type that is brought about from the inside, there is not yet a method of treatment for it.²⁶

Thus, in 1406, according to the authors' claim, there was an established therapy or therapies (the original language does not distinguish between singular and plural) for southern foot qi, but specific treatments for the northern type were still lacking.

Doctors remedied this perceived lack soon enough. By at least the mid-fifteenth century, references to northern styles of treatment began to crop up in the literature. The northern style, suited to hardier bodies, entailed vigorously draining qi in the manner of Zhang Congzheng. The evidence that qi was being drained was often in the diarrhea, vomiting, or sweating that the therapy induced. The southern style, à la Zhu Zhenheng, replenished healthy qi in the fragile body of a southerner, enabling that body to expel the nasty qi on its own. By the sixteenth century, as we will see in the next chapter, Li's theory that bad eating and drinking could cause foot qi had become the primary etiology that doctors discussed. The notion of northern and southern bodies and remedies continued to be prominent, but, in a newly reunified China, threatened by the rise of self-educated doctors touting region-specific expertise, elite physicians rejected this geographic factionalism and insisted on a unified universal medicine.

Li Gao's thirteenth-century theory is the first to present foot qi as diet induced, and most modern scholars, too, see historical foot qi as a dietary disease. But where Li implicates a diet of excess, one characterized by rich fatty foods and abundant wine, modern scholars insist that deficiency really caused it. Moreover, Li's ideas about northern and southern bodies are foreign to modern biomedical physicians' models of disease. Physicians today do not believe that the pores of people in south China are wider than those of the northern Chinese, and even if they did it would be irrelevant, as they do not suppose disease enters through the pores. Consequently, Li Gao's ideas, and the substantial literature that built on and responded to them in later centuries, are generally left out of histories of foot qi, ignored as a wrong turn in the road toward our present understanding. To exclude centuries of data because they do not conform to a narrative of progressive discovery—culminating in today's perfect understanding—is to take more interest in seeing our modern selves reflected than in comprehending what Chinese physicians and patients experienced and how they made sense of it. By taking Li's ideas seriously, as his contemporaries and generations of successors clearly did, we stand to gain a better understanding of how and why concepts of diet and constitution changed in China and how regional styles of medicine developed.

CHAPTER FIVE

Getting Rich and Getting Sick

In the mid-fifteenth century, an unfortunate gentleman suffering from foot qi found himself at the center of a dispute over appropriate therapy. Described by Dai Yuanli, the physician reporting the incident, as "fat and full," the patient had a form of foot qi that was relatively new in the context of China's long medical tradition. "Internal" foot qi, caused by overeating, had first been identified only about 200 years earlier. Dai describes his own therapeutic rationale:

> Because [the patient] ate fine, rich foods, slept with concubines, and endlessly indulged his desires, I judged that his essence (*jing*) and yin qi were both insufficient, and moisture and heat were too abundant, so I used essence and yin qi–augmenting [drugs] for his lower half and moisture and heat-clearing [drugs] for his upper half.[1]

Unfortunately, a meddlesome bystander observing this interaction failed to understand the subtlety of Dai's reasoning and scotched the treatment: "I gave him two formulas," reports Dai, "but someone said, 'With foot qi, you can't use a qi-replenishing method.' So he refused to take [the formulas]."[2] Dai then watched helplessly as the man was first treated with what Dai calls the "southern method," which appeared to have no effect, and then the "northern method," which involved strong purgatives. The latter proved somewhat too vigorous: the man died, Dai reports dryly, sitting on his chamber pot.[3]

This anecdote is an early example of two patterns apparent in medical literature of the sixteenth and seventeenth centuries: the growing prominence of a form of foot qi thought to be chronic and diet related and the contested transformation of this dietary disease from a regional to a universal disorder. Both patterns reflect the social and economic changes of China in the fourteenth through eighteenth centuries. This chapter examines why Li Gao's idea that overindulgence could cause foot qi, described in the previous chapter, became so prevalent at this time, and how its association with region weakened in some circles. In an age of rising prosperity and disintegrating social hierarchies, dietary foot qi—which started its life as a relatively minor form of the disease confined to northerners and non-Chinese—became the paradigmatic disease of excess, the signature disease of a rapidly commercializing empire.

Historians writing about foot qi have paid very little attention to this period, preferring to focus instead on the seventh through twelfth centuries. They imply that both the incidence of foot qi and innovations in understanding and treatment declined after the twelfth century. Some scholars emphasize aspects of medieval foot qi texts that seem to confirm a beriberi diagnosis while ignoring aspects that seem to contradict one, and others argue that those same texts could indicate other diagnoses.[4] But all alike give short shrift to late imperial sources. Why? Patients did not cease suffering from foot qi in the late imperial period. Though it is impossible to assess changes in incidence before the twentieth century, when statistical surveys and modern epidemiology emerged, case records published in the sixteenth century and later attest that many people experienced it then. Nor did doctors cease writing about it. Some of what they wrote, indeed, simply recapitulated what medieval authors had said about causes and cures, but much did not; ideas about internally caused foot qi were comparatively new. I suggest that these discussions have not garnered much attention because they fit poorly with the modern experience of beriberi. The dietary foot qi of sixteenth-century China afflicted comfortable people with sedentary lifestyles, whereas modern beriberi has appeared mostly among the poor and institutionalized. Moreover, the salient symptoms of rich man's foot qi resemble gout at least as closely as they do beriberi. Thus researchers determined to find a thiamine deficiency in premodern foot qi have marginalized sources from this period as less legitimately part of the disease's history. But who are we to say that the foot qi that late imperial doctors treated doesn't count? If they called it foot qi, it was foot qi. Better to try to understand it as they did. When we do that, we begin to see how the economic and social transformation of fifteenth- through nineteenth-century China influenced both health and the understanding of disease in this period.

Flaring Up: A Culture of Consumption Feeds a Chronic Disease

By the sixteenth century, a great deal had changed in China. The center of population had continued to shift south, driven by conflict in the north and drawn by opportunity. As it did so, the Chinese began to grow rich, and trade boomed. The fertile soil south of the Yangzi River supported a denser population than the north. The lakes and navigable rivers of the south, supplemented by canals, made transporting goods faster and cheaper than in the north, where there was relatively little water and the main river was the unmanageable Yellow. By the early sixteenth century, commerce was at the center of the southern economy; southern cities such as Suzhou had turned from backwaters into hubs of imperial and even world trade. Among the rich, a literature of connoisseurship sprang up, in which luxury goods were lovingly described in books with titles such as the *Treatise on Superfluous Things.*[5]

Ming dynasty literati were ambivalent about the new economy. They decried the explosion of commerce and decadent lifestyles, seeing them as a source of social decline. The increasing clout of merchants was a particular concern. Merchants stood on the bottom rung of the social ladder as defined by scholar-officials, deemed to contribute less to a functioning, harmonious society than the artisans, farmers, and (not coincidentally) scholar-officials who occupied the rungs above. Yet in the sixteenth century merchants were buying their way to respectability—meaning government positions. When a merchant family grew wealthy enough to spare a son or two from income-generating work, it would have sons educated for the imperial civil service exams so that they could compete for a place in officialdom. This was a strategy that had only recently become possible with the lifting of a ban on the sons and grandsons of merchants sitting for the exams.[6] Other merchant families bought their way in more directly, by purchasing titles outright from impoverished officials. Horrified officials attempted to reinforce the distinction between the merchant class and themselves by enacting sumptuary laws that forbade merchants from the kind of conspicuous consumption to which officials were entitled. These laws were more honored in the breach than in the observance, however. And at the same time as the Ming literati criticized the new opulence, they themselves enjoyed the fruits of expanded commerce, as Timothy Brook has shown; they took to new luxuries enthusiastically and in a spirit of competitive consumption.[7]

Among the objects most eagerly consumed and curated were books. After an initial decline in publishing and the book trade in the early Ming, by the sixteenth century publishing was a vibrant industry. The cost of printing plummeted, and the volume and diversity of commercial printing burgeoned, including medical treatises, formularies, books of materia medica, and cheap primers to facilitate studying medicine without a teacher. The relative abundance of sources is a boon for contemporary scholars; from the fifteenth century forward, we have more material to discipline our fantasy of what the past must have been like.[8] For historians of disease, the genre of collected case records that emerged in the sixteenth century is especially useful, showing doctors in action. Early case records are generally very simple, about a paragraph's worth of text, giving basic information about the patient's experience, from the initial complaint to the resolution, whether recovery (usually but not always) or death (very rarely). In between comes an account of the treatment, often including earlier therapies that failed. Such accounts had been sprinkled in earlier medical books as well, but in the sixteenth century books consisting entirely of case records, such as the *Stone Mountain Medical Case Histories* (*Shi shan yi an*) of 1520 or the *Categorized Case Records of Famous Doctors* (*Ming yi lei an*) of 1549, began to proliferate.[9] In encyclopedias of case records, editors incorporate examples from biographies and other writings of earlier periods, allowing us to see which historical cases they thought belonged together under the rubric of a single disease. They offer, in short, a rich reservoir of evidence about how doctors identified, classified, and treated disease and who suffered various kinds of diseases.

Literati physicians of the time, however, saw the increased availability of printed medical works as a mixed blessing. Suddenly more people had access to the objects that formed the basis of their authority, and it became more difficult to differentiate scholars from pretenders, the truly cultured from the merely entrepreneurial. Some healers even claimed to be members of famous medical lineages because they had acquired versions of the founders' books. In sum, for Chinese literati, and particularly for scholar-physicians, the late Ming was a time of great change and uncertainty. It was in this atmosphere of uncertainty that dietary foot qi became the prevalent concern in the foot qi literature.

By the sixteenth century, Li Gao's new form of foot qi, the kind caused by immoderate consumption, had become one of the types most written about in medical sources. The idea that internal accretion from unwise eating could cause the disease, novel in the twelfth century, had become commonplace, and many medical books were putting dietary foot qi on a par with, or even above, miasmatic foot qi as a disease of concern. Li Shizhen's *Systematic Materia Medica* (*Ben cao gang mu*, AD 1578), which is still the most-read work on materia medica in classical Chinese medicine, classifies the disease into four types: wind-and-wet, cold-and-wet, wet-and-hot, and food-accumulation.[10] Three of these recall the ancient etiology of invasive environmental qi, but the fourth follows the focus on diet and stasis that had emerged only a few centuries earlier.

There are at least two ways to account for the prominence of dietary foot qi in the medical literature of the sixteenth and seventeenth centuries. One is cultural and the other epidemiological, but both originate in the historical circumstances of rising wealth and commercialization in late Ming dynasty China. The cultural explanation for the increased concern about dietary foot qi is that it reflects unease or ambivalence about consumption among literati physicians. Some scholars have argued that as social status became more closely bound to wealth in the fifteenth and sixteenth centuries, classical physicians expressed anxiety about the change through their diagnoses. In her analysis of the case histories of Wang Ji (1463–1539), for example, Joanna Grant notes that Wang often identified excess in diet, drink, or sex as the cause of his male patients' illnesses, and she attributes this in part to Wang's own disapproval of rising merchant wealth in the region of south-central China where he lived.[11] Other classical physicians were also attuned to dietary indiscretion in this period. Discussions of diseases associated with poor digestion, stasis in the spleen and stomach systems, and "overnight food accumulation disorder" proliferate in the late imperial literature.

On the other hand, it may be that something *was* amiss in the eating and digestion of the patients whom scholar-physicians of this period were treating, and that their attention to dietary disorders reflects an epidemiological reality. There may have been at this time something like an epidemic of disorders in which an overly rich diet, drinking, and sedentary habits were implicated. Certainly the diet of the Ming elite was far from restrained. In addition, the symptoms and prognosis described in medical case records of this period resemble those of diseases associated with affluence and sedentary lifestyles in other times and places, such as gout or diabetes. Let us examine late imperial foot qi as the case records described it.

One striking and consistent feature of the dietary foot qi that doctors were treating in this period was that it was a chronic, recurring condition. Early literature had been divided on whether foot qi was chronic or acute. The most famous early sources—Sun Simiao's and Chao Yuanfang's, which we have examined in earlier chapters—tended to emphasize the disease's lethality and the importance of correcting the dysfunction for good. Sun, in fact, suggested that recurrence was actually a sign of faulty treatment. He cautioned that if a doctor did not use moxibustion and drugs together, he would leave the patient "half cured and half dead, so that even one who has recovered may experience another outbreak within one or two years."[12]

Others, however, including Sun's near-contemporary Su Jing, accepted recurrence as characteristic of the disease, not an indication that the healer was inferior. Su wrote that "no foot qi sufferer can be cured permanently. As soon as spring and summer arrive, the illness will once again break out."[13] Others agreed. Xu Sigong observed that "foot qi is not like other diseases; once one has suffered foot qi, it is hard to recover and easy to experience a flare-up."[14] For his part, Su wrote as if living with the disease were possible and bearable given the right strategies for managing it. To doctors, he offered this recommendation: "It is advisable to drain the qi three to five times per month. Regularly administer drugs, from time to time draining qi and from time to time drawing sweat."[15] The patient, he additionally suggests, should keep a supply of appropriate drugs on hand. "Foot qi sufferers, whether roaming about or at home, always need to have Gold Sprouts (*jin ya*) and Purple Snow (*zi xue*) nearby."[16] This sounds more like an asthmatic keeping an inhaler at hand than a strategy for dealing with a progressive, fatal disease.

By the sixteenth century recurrence was a standard feature of new foot qi literature. Medical authors used the terms *fa*, *fa dong*, and *fu zuo*, any of which might in this context be translated "manifests," "breaks out," or "acts up," to express this aspect of the disease. In his AD 1515 *Orthodox Transmission of Medical Knowledge* (*Yi xue zheng chuan*), Yu Tuan wrote, "Sometimes after ten days, or half a month, [the symptoms] will recur just as before . . . In most cases like this, the patient has foot qi."[17] Among the sufferers described in *Categorized Case Records of Famous Doctors* is the monk Pu Qing, who "suffered this [that is, foot qi] for twenty years. Each time it broke out, during the first two months, he would use moxibustion" to stop the pain. An unnamed person of Shangzhou[18] is described as not having walked in decades. For another unnamed sufferer, the disease would "flare up seasonally and become unbearable." To control the pain, he burned moxa above the ankle—on the inside of the ankle if the pain was on the inside, and on the outside if it was on the outside.[19]

This last detail highlights one consequence of perceiving foot qi as a chronic disease: for many, the main concern was not how to eradicate it but how to manage its tendency to break out painfully.

Accordingly, one sees many management strategies in the late imperial medical literature: washes and rinses meant to be applied daily over a long period, poultices for dealing with severe outbreaks, and drugs to be taken prophylactically in the seasons when symptoms are most likely to recur. The author of *Secretly-Transmitted Essential Oral Formulas for Diagnosing and Treating* (*Mi chuan zheng zhi yao jue*) of 1441 recommends Wet-Expelling Decoction and Papaya Pills, noting that "these formulas are both suitable for regular use." If these formulas don't take care of the occasional outbreak, he offers another solution. "When foot qi flares up, and your feet are in intolerable pain, take Five-Ingredient Powder. Add three to five whole scorpions, put the mixture in wine, and decoct."[20] The author of the AD 1575 *Introduction to the Study of Medicine* (*Yi xue ru men*) informs us that Leg-Replacement Pills have a similar prophylactic function: "Regularly taking [Leg-Replacement Pills] loosens up the sinews and lightens the feet, [ensuring that] you will never suffer from foot qi." He also recommends eating raw chestnuts, ten or so daily.[21]

Many of the sixteenth-century authors mention exercises and external therapies, such as taking an evening constitutional and applying foot washes. Take this formula from the AD 1550 *Excellent Formulas for Rescuing People in Emergency Situations* (*Ji jiu liang fang*), for example:

> Every night rub salt on your legs and knees down to your toenails. Leave it to sink in for a little while, and then use hot water to soak and wash the legs, and [the symptoms] will not recur. Once there was a person with foot qi, for whom all of the various formulas were ineffective. [Later] he got hold of this formula, and regularly used it, steeping and soaking, and [foot qi] did not break out again.[22]

The author does not say that the patient was cured. Although the classical doctor's ideal may have been to cure, many medical authors accepted that, for this disease, it was more feasible to prevent and manage the recurrence of symptoms instead.

In addition to highlighting foot qi's chronicity, the case histories of this period also emphasize symptoms in the legs and feet and rarely mention the vomiting, panting, dementia, and heart palpitations that seventh-century writers had warned about.[23] Pain, particularly in the feet and legs, was the symptom most commonly associated with foot qi in the late imperial period. Many sources refer to the "unbearable pain" of the sufferer, and some describe the attendant swelling in colorful terms such as "the feet and calves are swollen like melons and gourds."[24] Even the names of the most commonly cited drug formulas indicate which symptoms sufferers most urgently craved relief for, and what kind of debility they most wanted their physicians to resolve. One of the most popular formulas, for example, was Angelica Plucking-Out-the-Pain Decoction (*dang gui nian tong tang*). Another was Spring-in-Your-Step Decoction (*jian bu tang*), with such variations on the theme as Flying-Steps-of-an-Immortal Pills (*shen xian fei bu wan*) and Foot-Lightening Pills (*qing jiao wan*). Equally popular were Leg-Replacement Pills (*huan tui wan*), which had originally appeared in the *Pharmacy Formulary* of AD 1080. A later author explains their effect: "In the past, when I had this illness [that is, foot qi], I took this formula for one month. My foot strength was immediately restored. The formula has the function of replacing your legs [with healthy ones]."[25] None of these plaintively named formulas appeared before the eleventh century.

Sometimes an author indicates that he considers foot qi to be primarily a pain disorder by placing it among other such ailments in his books. In *Restoring Health from the Myriad Diseases* [literally, "Returning to springtime from the myriad diseases"] (*Wan bing hui chun*, 1587), for example, foot qi appears in the same chapter as "head pain," "belly pain," "lower back pain," and "back pain." Although the term *foot qi* lacks the *tong* that signifies pain, its inclusion in this chapter suggests that the author considers foot qi analogous to pain in other parts of the body.[26]

Medical case records, too, overwhelmingly emphasize swelling and pain in the extremities. Out of the twenty-nine cases that the *Categorized Case Records of Famous Doctors* (1549) identifies as foot qi, twenty-one name foot swelling, pain, inability to walk, or a combination of these three as the disease's primary symptoms. The descriptions are vivid: one patient's foot pain is "like being struck by arrows," whereas another's is "like a weapon stabbing" her. A third found that his lower legs swelled up "like pillars" when the disease manifested. So intense was the pain for one man that he "could not stand to wear shoes" and rode his horse barefoot, letting the stirrups hang down and controlling the horse's movement with a bamboo switch instead of his feet.[27] Nor was the pain always confined to the feet and lower legs. Late imperial foot qi also involved pain and swelling in the hands and fingers, symptoms that had never featured in earlier descriptions of the disease. As the *Universal Aid Formulary* pointed out in 1406, "The kind that is brought about from the inside [that is, 'internal injury' foot qi] sometimes reaches the hands and fingers."[28] Several of the cases included in the *Categorized Case Records of Famous Doctors* also refer to painful symptoms in the hands.[29]

Debilitating pain manifesting in the feet, the hands, and other joints, flaring up and remitting over the course of years or decades and associated with sedentary lifestyles and rich diets—this late imperial variety of foot qi bears a strong resemblance to today's gout. Gout is an extremely painful condition that is difficult to manage. Its main symptoms, according to a contemporary biochemistry textbook, are

> episodes of severe acute joint pain and swelling (particularly in the great toe, midfoot, ankle, and knee). These episodes tend to resolve completely and spontaneously within a week even without treatment. If not properly treated, however, this acute, self-limited form of the disease can evolve over many years into a chronic, destructive pattern resulting in more frequent and sustained periods of pain and resultant joint deformity.[30]

Inside the gouty body, an excess of uric acid in the blood forms crystals, which tend to accumulate at the joints. The patient's body, doing what a responsible body does in reaction to injury, inflames the surrounding skin, and this doubles the pain the patient feels. Sometimes the piles of crystals form tophi, stonelike deposits that push their way through the skin in the form of white, chalky excretions. In general it is best to refrain from retrospective diagnoses, and even if some cases of foot qi described in this period were what a doctor today would identify as gout, that would not indicate that all foot qi in history (or all "real" foot qi in history) was actually gout. But the similarities are certainly suggestive, and they make it all the more clear how foot qi's modern translation into beriberi has obscured other possibilities and potentially other applications for classical medical knowledge.

From Region to Class: Reasserting the Universal Canon

As chronic dietary foot qi was becoming more prominent in the gilded age of late Ming China, it was losing its original association with region. It was becoming instead a disease that afflicted people across the empire. In fact, the north–south distinction came under attack by prominent physicians who asserted that neither the internal nor the external form of foot qi was regionally bounded. It was perfectly evident, they argued, that economic status and lifestyle varied dramatically within a single region and that no region was free of pernicious environmental qi; one might therefore encounter "northern" and "southern" types in the very same location.

We see the argument beginning to develop in the anecdote with which this chapter began. Dai Yuanli was a southerner who counted himself a disciple of Zhu Zhenheng; as the previous chapter showed, Zhu's qi-replenishing method came to be perceived as a characteristically southern style of therapy. Nevertheless, in this anecdote Dai presents region-based recommendations and prohibitions as rigid and rote. The "someone" whose doubts moved the patient to refuse Dai's treatment saw in Dai's proposed formulas "a qi-replenishing method" (*bu fa*) and believed there was a blanket prohibition on treating foot qi with such a method, associated with the south. But Dai makes it clear that he was not reflexively offering a "southern" therapy and simply pulling a qi-replenishing formula out of a readymade tool kit. He combined qi-boosting drugs with heat-clearing drugs to address this individual's unique combination of deficiency (jing and yin qi) and excess (heat and moisture). The competing doctors who replace him, on the other hand, and whose advice quickly kills the patient, use the "southern method" and the "northern method." Perceiving illness and healing through a regional lens has facilitated a narrow sectarian form of clinical reasoning that fails to grasp the larger picture.

Later writers amplified this sort of critique. In *The Systematic Study of Medicine* (*Yi xue gang mu*, 1565), Lou Ying wrote, "According to what people say, it is not necessary to use north and south to distinguish hot and cold [types of foot qi]. Not all externally contracted [cases involving] cold and wet qi are southern. Not all internal-injury [cases involving] wine are northern."[31] Zhang Jiebin, one of the most influential doctors of his day, framed it as a rhetorical question in 1636: "In the north there is also cold and wet qi [that is, qi that can infect people from the outside], and do southerners really imbibe less of the wet qi of wine [than northerners]? Thus the distinction certainly is not always between northern and southern types."[32] And in a mid-sixteenth-century discussion, the author explains thoughtfully:

> Even though the north lacks low places, external wetness due to braving rain and dew also occurs there. Even if the south lacks dairy foods, inner wetness due to fish, meat, melons and fruits also occurs there. One can see that both north and south have internal and external wet [qi]. It is best to differentiate by following the signs [that is, symptoms]. You cannot use region exclusively to limit (the diagnosis).[33]

For writers such as these, northern foot qi, which in the thirteenth century had reflected literate doctors' interest in and anxiety about north–south difference, came to mean simply internal foot qi, a kind of dietary disease with no regional inflection.

The rejection of northern and southern foot qi was part of a broader backlash against the idea of regional types of therapy. This backlash did not entail rejecting techniques that physicians had previously understood as regional therapies but rather relabeling them. For example, Li Zhongzi (1588–1655) argued that Zhang Congzheng's "attacking and purging" style—which had been seen as the signature of aggressive northern therapy, suited to northern climates and conditions—was appropriate for Zhang's patients not because they were northerners but because they were simple hardworking people. As Li explained: "The patients Zhang Congzheng cured were poor and ignoble so they could withstand his drastic purgatives."[34] He contrasted Zhang with Xue Ji (1487–1559), whose use of warming and replenishing medications had identified him—as much as the fact that he was a southerner—as a proponent of the southern style of therapy. Paralleling his judgment of Zhang's clientele and their socioeconomic status, Li explained, "The patients Xue Ji cured were mainly the wealthy and noble so they were well suited to his restoratives."[35]

This shift in emphasis to social and economic status and away from differences between Chinese and non-Chinese, southern and northern cultures, reflects ways in which the Chinese physician's world had changed by the sixteenth century. The empire was once again under Han Chinese rule and had been so for 200 years. The caste system that the Mongols had enforced in the thirteenth and fourteenth centuries, which gave non-Chinese different privileges and rights from Chinese and ranked northern Chinese above southern Chinese, no longer obtained. Distinctions between Chinese and non-Chinese bodies and habits were a less persistent concern than they had been in Li Gao's time. In this setting, what mattered more than region was class. The greatest threat to the status of educated Chinese elite was no longer non-Han peoples and their barbarian ways, but the increasing fluidity of the social hierarchy. Both upward and downward social mobility were accelerating.

For physicians in particular, the new social mobility meant that the medical marketplace was more diverse and competitive than it had been before. One reason was the increased difficulty of passing the civil service exams and of entering officialdom through that route. More and more literate candidates sat for the civil service examinations, but the number of official positions available was not increasing nearly as quickly, so an ever-larger pool of degree holders found themselves without government employment. Many failed examination candidates turned to respectable second-choice careers such as medicine to support themselves or make their names, causing an influx of educated physicians from among the ranks of the elite. There was a similar influx from below because of the printing and publishing boom, which expanded access to the main source of scholar-physicians' authority: books.[36]

The scholar-physicians who opposed the idea of regionally bounded foot qi thus were expressing more than just a general concern about rising wealth and immoderate consumption. They were also concerned about how claims that particular schools of therapy suited particular regions undercut the idea of universal expertise based on the classics, especially the *Inner Canon*. In his *Standards for Diagnosis and Therapy* (*Zheng zhi zhun sheng*, 1602) the physician Wang Kentang harshly criticizes the northern and southern currents of interpretation (*xue pai*) that have developed as a result of what he considers a muddled understanding of Li Gao's theory:

> According to Dongyuan's [that is, Li Gao's] discussion of southern foot qi, externally contracted cold and wet qi should be treated with cooling medicines, while "northern" foot qi—in other words internally-caused damage from wine and milk—should be treated with wet and hot drugs. This filled in a spot that previous doctors had missed [that is, treatment for internal foot qi]. Later scholars muddled [this teaching], and there developed two factions, a northern and a southern one, each maligning the other. The southerners criticize the northern faction, saying that what they discuss is a northern illness, and what they use to treat it is a northern method, which will not work in the south. The northern faction criticizes the southern faction, saying that what they discuss is a southern illness, and what they use is a southern method, which will not work in the north. Alas! They set up new theories, and don't investigate the *Inner Canon*'s teachings from head to tail. They always invent these names, in order to make later people stick to their teachings. Knowing the first [type] but not the second, they are both mistaken.[37]

Wang's reference to the *Inner Canon* is telling. He attacks the north–south distinction, and the northern and southern "schools" that had emerged, to reassert the universal wisdom of the ancient medical canon. From his perspective, the regional factions imparted only fragments of medical knowledge and distracted young doctors from mastering the *Inner Canon* and the *Treatise on Cold Damage Disorders*, from which a good doctor's power and authority came. In Wang Kentang's case, we might well read his promotion of a universal and authoritative system of medicine as an extension of his personal investment in a universal and authoritative system of government. Not only did Wang himself serve in a series of high government posts after passing the top-level civil service examination in 1589, but his grandfather and father had likewise held high official positions after succeeding in the examination system. His career and family background likely influenced the way in which Wang approached the increasingly diverse medical literature proliferating in his day. In fact, from the sixteenth century on, insistence on northern and southern foot qi, or insistence that there was no such difference, generally reflects the author's status. The most politically powerful, highest-status physicians such as Wang Kentang tended to see regional diseases as bogus and regional therapies as illegitimate; they reasserted the primacy of the universal medical canon and, by implication, of a unified culture under a central government. It was the less eminent—from an official perspective—who were more likely to preserve and elaborate on the north–south distinction that Li Gao had outlined in the thirteenth century and to distinguish themselves as specialists in regional medicine. These constituted different strategies for attaining recognition in a crowded field.

* * *

In the sixteenth century, more and more elite scholar-physicians wrote about foot qi as a disease of excess consumption, representative of a whole class of consumption-related diseases that attained new prominence in this period. Although diet-induced foot qi had first appeared in medical literature 300 years earlier, at that time its significance had been rather different. Originally, dietary foot qi had highlighted the differences between northerners and southerners, between Han Chinese and non-Chinese, during a period of political division. But by the 1500s, Li Gao's "northern" foot qi had become universal, at least in the writing of literati physicians. Changing a commonly discussed disease from a regional disorder into a universal one was a way for elite scholar-physicians to preserve their authority by insisting on the unity of medical knowledge and may also have been a way of expressing their disapproval and anxiety about the increasingly robust connection between wealth and power in the Chinese empire. But the cultural explanation alone is insufficient and too cynical; in part, probably, the sixteenth-century rise of dietary foot qi really does reflect changes in diet and epidemiology. This was, after all, a time of conspicuous consumption, including the type of conspicuous consumption that is still most valued in Chinese culture: that of the banquet table.

Ironically, the next major shift in foot qi's meaning, analyzed in the following chapter, would transform it from a dietary disorder associated mostly with the affluent into beriberi, a vitamin deficiency disorder associated with the poor and institutionalized. Neither gout nor beriberi, of course, is a more natural or correct meaning for this disease name. In each setting, physicians applied an old and commonly used name to a condition prominent among their patients. But the differences between the foot qi of the sixteenth century and that of the early twentieth should give us pause and help to place beriberi in its proper perspective. Although scholars today tend to see it as the true identity of foot qi, beriberi is just one biomedical disease among many that foot qi has signified, and it is just as redolent of its particular time and social context as other biomedical equivalents we might propose for foot qi in different periods.

CHAPTER SIX

Creating Beriberi in Meiji Japan

In this chapter we turn to Japan. It was there that, in the late nineteenth and early twentieth centuries, a new meaning for foot qi emerged. Practitioners of Western medicine came to view *kakke*—the Japanese pronunciation of foot qi—as a disease caused by ingesting too little of a micronutrient, thiamine. Because biomedicine predominates in most societies today, it can be more difficult to see how this reinterpretation of foot qi reflects the political, economic, and social circumstances that surrounded its emergence than it was to see how imperial politics in China produced northern and southern foot qi in the early modern period, or bureaucratic foot qi in the eleventh century. Authoritative sources tell us that beriberi is not just *a* meaning of *kakke* but *the* meaning, the correct understanding of the old term in all times and places. But this chapter shows that *kakke*-as-beriberi is every bit as much an artifact of its time—the setting in which it first appeared—as northern foot qi and bureaucratic foot qi are artifacts of theirs.

Beriberi, now rare, is a deficiency of dietary vitamin B1, also called thiamine. In instances where a person's diet is so limited or regimented that it does not provide enough thiamine—historically, this has occurred most often in institutional settings such as the military or hospitals, or in times of famine—the symptoms of the disorder will appear over the course of six to eight weeks. It might manifest in sharp and aching pain as the victim's nerves deteriorate; it might produce high blood pressure, swelling in the extremities, and chest pain; if allowed to develop unchecked, it generally ends in heart failure. Many foods contain thiamine and can help prevent beriberi. Spinach, peas, lentils, pork, wheat germ, milk, oranges, and many kinds of nuts are rich in the vitamin. Brown rice also provides enough thiamine to prevent the illness. Raw-fish eaters and alcoholics are at a disadvantage, the former because fish contain a thiamine-destroying enzyme that is only deactivated once the fish is cooked, and the latter because they tend to consume calories in the form of alcohol, at the expense of other nutrients.[1] But, generally, given an even moderately varied diet, beriberi is easy to avoid.

Histories of beriberi in the late nineteenth and early twentieth centuries have tended to be celebratory in tone, holding up the elucidation of the disease's cause as a landmark in medical progress.[2] For decades, scientists around the world struggled to understand beriberi. The predominance of germ theory and the successful identification of numerous disease-causing microbes in the 1880s may have complicated the struggle; when all the world's illnesses seemed traceable to the presence of microscopic bugs, few suspected that the absence of a micronutrient could debilitate and kill just as surely.[3] By the 1910s, however, after many failed efforts to identify the "beriberi germ," the international scientific community finally came to a consensus that beriberi was instead caused by eating too little of a newly discovered object, soon to be known as a vitamin.[4] After this, armed with the vitamin deficiency disorder as a new diagnostic category, doctors began to look for other ailments that might fit into it. One by one, chronic dietary deficiencies began to fall into line: scientists soon understood the etiology of scurvy, rickets, and pellagra. With the synthesis of vitamins in the 1910s and 1920s, nutritional deficiency disorders became gratifyingly easy to prevent and treat, at least on a technical level (the social and economic factors at the root of malnutrition have proven intractable). This accomplishment is often overshadowed by the contemporaneous bacteriological revolution that ultimately yielded antibiotics, but the nutrition-science revolution was equally profound. It ushered in what Rima Apple has called "vitamania," changing the way people ate and thought about eating and improving their resistance to and recovery from infectious diseases. And it all started with beriberi.[5] Kenneth J. Carpenter best summarizes this perspective:

> This *is* a success story: the puzzle . . . was finally solved, and beriberi was found to result from a lack of something required in seemingly infinitesimal quantities. Our present knowledge required the contributions of people from different specialties: physicians, pathologists, epidemiologists, chemists, physiologists, nutritionists, and biochemists, and also chemical engineers in the pharmaceutical industry.[6]

This is an accurate summation as far as it goes. The tortuous paths that led, between the 1870s and the 1930s, to the discovery of vitamins, the elucidation of conditions caused by their absence, and their synthesis in the lab do make a thrilling "medical detective story," as Carpenter writes.[7] Because in Japan the late nineteenth century beriberi epidemics were seen as epidemics of *kakke*, once scientists understood correctly what had caused them, "thiamine deficiency" superseded all older understandings of the term *kakke*. From the triumphant perspective articulated in the preceding paragraph, this seems like progress: thiamine deficiency was the correct understanding of the disease, and it finally swept away confused older concepts.

This chapter argues, however, that the story of how *kakke* acquired its modern dictionary definition is one of creation rather than discovery. Doctors in the nineteenth century did not discover that *kakke* is a nutritional deficiency disorder. Instead, faced with an extraordinary epidemic and armed with the tools of late nineteenth-century medicine, they redefined *kakke* as a nutritional deficiency disorder, creating a new category of disease in the process. The Japanese government's efforts to modernize following a Western model supplied the conditions necessary for this development. The modernization of the Japanese military brought about the epidemiological conditions, producing Asia's largest-scale beriberi outbreaks. Reforms of the health care and educational systems created the epistemological conditions, making Western-style physicians and scientists the authorities qualified to investigate public health problems. When we look at the redefinition of *kakke* as the product of the peculiar epidemiological, intellectual, social, and economic circumstances of the time, the story is more complicated, the conclusion less triumphant, and the definition less absolute than historians have typically suggested.

Beriberi, a Disease of Western Expansion

It is tempting to think of beriberi as a timeless condition of the pre-modern world; human bodies have likely responded in a similar way to vitamin deficits regardless of whether they occurred a hundred years ago or a thousand years ago. And indeed, classic accounts of disease history such as William McNeill's *Plagues and Peoples* and Thomas McKeown's *The Role of Medicine* suggest that malnutrition was a characteristic condition of human existence from the agricultural revolution of 10,000 years ago to the dawn of the modern age.[8] But beriberi is really a signature disease of the nineteenth and early twentieth centuries. In this sense it resembles (and probably contributed to mortality from) cholera and tuberculosis, "modern epidemics" of diseases that, although presumably present earlier in history, flourished particularly in industrializing cities and highlighted patterns of transportation, settlement, and labor that were new.[9] Likewise, although clinical nutritional deficiencies historically may have emerged anytime there was a prolonged siege or famine, it was not until the age of imperialism that they became a feature of regular peacetime life for many people. One might reasonably refer to them as imperial epidemics.

The earliest appearances of the word *beriberi* in a Western language suggest its connection to expanding empires, showing that, like scurvy, it became prominent as sea voyages grew longer and more ambitious. The term first appeared in Portuguese in the sixteenth century and likely derives from a language of South Asia, but today its true etymology is anything but certain. The current *Oxford English Dictionary* asserts confidently that the word is a doubling of the Sinhalese *beri*, citing an eighteenth-century European travel narrative as its earliest appearance in the English language. But that asserted origin is questionable; already in the nineteenth century, confusion clouded the issue. The German scientist Heinrich Botho Scheube catalogued proposed etymologies for *beriberi* derived from Hindi, Sinhalese, and

Arabic words meaning everything from "weakness" to "sailor" to "rapid breathing" to "swelling" and even "sheep," the latter thought to reflect the victim's sheeplike gait![10] Most philologists and scientists interested in the origins of the term confessed to the kind of uncertainty that Edward Vedder expressed in his 1913 book *Beriberi*: "It is impossible to definitely trace the origin of the word beriberi, but it is undoubtedly an oriental word and probably from some language allied to or derived from Malay."[11]

These conjectures about the origins of the term suggest two things about the disease that it labels: first, that the European adventurers who wrote about it had not seen it before, and encountered it for the first time in Asia. But second—and just as important for our purposes—they also suggest that it was unfamiliar to the people whom those adventurers encountered. Most of the beriberi victims that the Western literature of the seventeenth century discusses were Europeans, not natives. The Portuguese historian Diogo do Couto wrote in 1568 of his experience in India, "Our people sickened of a disease called berbere, the belly and legs swell, and in a few days they die, as there died many, ten or twelve a day." Another observer, writing in 1659, noted that the disease was common in parts of India and Ceylon (now Sri Lanka), but "it does not vex the natives so much as foreigners." In *The Fatal History of Portuguese Ceylon*, written in 1685, Joao Ribeiro reported, "The Portuguese in the Island suffer from another sickness which the natives call béri-béri."[12] One can imagine how the Portuguese sailors, after months at sea or as a result of failing to adjust to the local diet, might have begun to show signs of extreme nutritional deficiency. But *beriberi*, whether derived from Sinhalese, Hindi, or "some language allied to or derived from Malay," seems to have been more an ad hoc description of the foreigners' symptoms than a fixed category of disease among the peoples of South and Southeast Asia. Indeed, in 1835, an English Orientalist declared, "As to the appellation Beriberi, it appears to me perfectly unaccountable how it could ever have crept into such general use as it has; for it is perfectly unintelligible to the Natives from whom it is said to have originated."[13] Had it been a disease category of long standing—as foot qi was in East Asia—one would expect the term *beriberi* to have elicited recognition among Indians in the early nineteenth century and to have a place in traditional medical literature.

Instead, it was not until the late nineteenth century that beriberi became more familiar to the native peoples of Asia themselves. Sixty percent of the Javanese soldiers serving in a Dutch army unit in Sumatra in 1886 developed beriberi, whereas very few of their European counterparts did. Beriberi afflicted indentured sugarcane laborers in the South Pacific. It hobbled the native labor force in the U.S.-occupied Philippines in the early twentieth century. And the Japanese suffered some of the worst beriberi epidemics of all—in 1895, as Japan set up its new colony in Taiwan, some 95 percent of its occupying army fell victim to the disease.[14]

Western observers, informed by social Darwinist-inflected ideas about race and nation, began to view beriberi as a disease to which the people of East Asia were particularly prone. This contradicted the earlier experience of beriberi-stricken Europeans but reflected the reality at the time, when victims were disproportionately Asian. Albrecht Wernich opined in 1877, "People of Japanese descent have a disposition for *kakké*."[15] In 1906, Edouard Jeanselme listed "la race" as the primary "predisposing cause" for beriberi, writing, "The facility with which the Japanese, the Chinese, and the Malays contract beriberi is really surprising. Hygienic and alimentary conditions are powerless to explain this morbid tendency; one must admit a truly ethnic receptivity [to the disease]."[16] As the historian David Arnold has noted, "In the racialized discourse of late nineteenth- and early twentieth-century tropical medicine it was typically on the Chinese body that beriberi was inscribed."[17] This was ironic, given how much more widespread it was in Japan than in China, but reinforced the emerging idea that China was the Sick Man of Asia, embedding sickliness as part of an "increasingly racialized Chinese identity," a process that Larissa N. Heinrich has traced in detail.[18] When the Far Eastern Association of Tropical Medicine (FEATM) concluded in 1910, at the end of its first congress, that beriberi was a disease caused by diet, they did not explicitly mention race; nevertheless, their resolution condemned a dietary pattern presumed to be timelessly characteristic of Asian races: "Beriberi is associated with the continuous consumption of white (polished) rice, as the staple article of diet."[19] As Michael Worboys has shown in Western surveys of colonial malnutrition, the emphasis on foolish native habits "allowed evidence of the recent origins of the problem to be ignored."[20]

The international elite represented in the FEATM was unaware that polished rice had become the staple diet of ordinary Asians only recently; before the nineteenth century all but the very wealthiest relied on mixed grains or brown rice. If the first phase of beriberi's spread had reflected the increasingly ambitious sea voyages of Europeans, this second phase was the consequence of dietary changes of the nineteenth century connected, in most cases, to new relationships of dependency and control. As European nations and Japan began to consolidate their power in Asia, patterns of food production and processing changed. In Japan and in European colonies in Asia, many farmers stopped producing their own rice, and instead rice was brought to a central location, processed, and redistributed. The mills that processed it, starting in 1855 and accelerating thereafter, were modern factories where rice was hulled by steam-powered machines.[21] Steam milling stripped the rice of its bran, and the nutrients contained therein, much more thoroughly than hand pounding had done, and this made previously expensive white rice cheaply available. The poorest people, unable to afford much more than rice, were subsisting on a diet more nutrient-poor than ever before.

One example of the mechanics of this shift is the U.S.-occupied Philippines in the early twentieth century. There, rice farmers who had previously grown their own food, and even exported some grain, switched to cash crops like tobacco and sugarcane. The government began importing rice from Saigon to feed its no longer self-sufficient peasants. The rice was thoroughly hulled and refined in Saigon before being loaded onto a boat for the Philippines; without its bran, rice was lighter and took up less room, so more white than brown rice could be shipped for the same cost. Refined rice was also less prone to rot or animal infestation than brown rice, so it was better suited to being shipped long distances. Refined rice was not, however, able to provide adequate amounts of thiamine. The result was that beriberi soon joined malaria, cholera, smallpox, and tuberculosis as a top killer of poor Filipinos.[22] As the example of the Philippines suggests, these changes in processing and distribution most affected marginal populations, those whose diet choices were constrained either by regulations or by poverty.

Accompanying these changes in the distribution and nutritional quality of food were equally important changes in the way governments perceived epidemics. Before the late nineteenth century, an epidemic among the poor was a governmental concern only to the extent that the illness's survivors might sink into desperation and rebel. As governments began to build colonies far from the metropole, however, they relied more and more on their subjects as tools to expand and maintain empires. Their subjects' health therefore became a crucial element in determining their utility to the state. Governments worried in particular about keeping soldiers healthy because the expansion and stability of colonial possessions depended on military might. But the health of ordinary citizens also attracted bureaucrats' attention: factory owners, public health organizations, and government agencies began to track workers' health and tabulate days of work, and amounts of profit, lost to illness. Military and prison doctors could track patients' symptoms and habits; hospital officials recorded the course of each patient's illness and compiled admission and mortality data. At a time when new structures of political and economic power were bringing about beriberi epidemics on an unprecedented scale, new systems for recording and organizing data made the parameters of epidemics visible. These factors converged to make beriberi prominent.[23]

Beriberi was a particularly acute administrative problem because of its effects on imperial armies. The disease often felled more soldiers or sailors than enemy weapons did, and it stymied colonial governments' efforts to control the populations they governed. Learning more about its cause and treatment therefore became a governmental priority, and the most important beriberi research was done under state sponsorship. The Dutch government organized the Pekelharing Commission in the 1880s, sending its top scientists to the colony of Java to investigate beriberi there. Robert Williams, the American who first succeeded in synthesizing vitamin B1 in 1925, had begun investigating beriberi at the American-run Bureau of Science in the Philippines. And the Meiji government in Japan also devoted considerable resources to the problem, establishing a hospital devoted to researching and treating beriberi.

Thus a disease that had first attracted attention among European adventurers at the beginning of the age of exploration rose, by the apex of the age of imperialism, to become a central preoccupation in the new field of tropical medicine. Putatively beriberi—along with malaria, yellow fever, plague, and a host of others—was a "tropical disease," its incidence mostly confined to tropical latitudes and climates.[24] As scholars have recently pointed out, these diseases are not, in fact, so bounded by geography; malaria has afflicted people in northern Europe and Siberia, yellow fever was a notorious scourge in eighteenth-century Philadelphia, and plague at different times has decimated populations in Western Europe and Manchuria.[25] As for beriberi, the Japanese islands and neighboring Korea, where thousands of soldiers came down with the disease during the Russo-Japanese War, were clearly not tropical. But designating some ailments "tropical diseases" gave them the appearance of permanence, implied that they inhered in relatively unchanging characteristics of a place or a people. The label obscured the extent to which the distribution of these diseases reflected patterns of privilege and poverty and the ways in which those patterns had been changing globally. Filing beriberi under "tropical disease" contributed to the narrative that the world outside of Europe was—had always been—sick, and that white men were tasked with the burden of curing it.[26] In Japan, the existence of an ancient corpus of medical literature helped to reinforce the notion that this particular "tropical disease" inhered in the place. But as we shall see in the next section, the content of Japanese sources suggests otherwise.

In Japan between the seventeenth and twentieth centuries, two waves of *kakke* are visible. In each, political and economic change brought disability and death to a segment of the population, and concomitant intellectual change shaped the way doctors understood that suffering. But the political and economic circumstances that precipitated the first wave, beginning in the seventeenth century, differed from those that brought on the second, beginning in the late nineteenth century, and so did the intellectual milieu that informed doctors' perspectives. What had been a disease of the comfortable, sedentary classes in eighteenth-century Japan, associated with peace and rising prosperity, became a disease of military conscripts and impoverished students in the late nineteenth century, associated with Japan's rapid modernization on a Western model. Doctors interpreted the earlier *kakke* through the lens of classical Sino-Japanese medicine and the later *kakke* through the lens of Western medicine. The later *kakke* became archetypal and still colors views of disease and medicine in East Asian history. Here, we will examine each of these waves of disease in turn, to understand them in the context of their time.

The Emergence of Japanese *Kakke*

In Japan before the nineteenth century, *kakke* often resembled the diseases indicated by the same two characters in Chinese medical texts: they were chronic, recurring afflictions of the well-to-do whose symptoms varied. This is not surprising given that, like many other classical terms, foot qi (*kakke*) was originally imported to Japan from China, and much of the early Japanese literature on the disease consisted of compilations of Chinese sources. The teachings and practices of classical Chinese medicine reached Japan by the sixth century, and in subsequent centuries its influence grew.[27] When the fledgling Japanese government sent delegations to the continent in the seventh through ninth centuries, medical knowledge was one of the resources that they sought to acquire. Japanese doctors were trained in the same therapeutic classics as Chinese doctors. This is not to deny that Japanese physicians innovated using these tools; we have records of Japanese drug formularies as early as AD 808, and doctors produced many important medical books in their own right.[28] But the foundations of Japanese medical practice lay in China. Japanese medical literature, mostly written in classical Chinese, was for a long time virtually indistinguishable from the literature produced by Chinese doctors. Even the name for traditional medicine in Japan reflects its Chinese origins: *kampō*, "Han [Chinese] formulas."[29]

It is therefore unsurprising that before the nineteenth century *kakke* in Japanese treatises was nearly identical to foot qi in Chinese ones. Books such as the ninth-century *Formulas at the Heart of Medicine* (*Ishimpō*), produced in Japan, include discussions of *kakke* that are today unique, but that is only because they were not preserved in China; Chinese doctors wrote them. *Kakke* occasionally appeared in a unique context in Japan, such as in medieval treatises on wound medicine, produced during a period of frequent warfare.[30] But, for the most part, later books quoted the material in the *Formulas at the Heart of Medicine* and the *Formulas Worth a Thousand in Gold* by the Chinese author Sun Simiao.

This began to change in the eighteenth through early nineteenth centuries, when many new books on *kakke* emerged in Japan. A disease that formerly occupied only scattered corners of Japanese medical collections suddenly became the sole focus of at least two dozen specialty treatises.[31] Something had made *kakke* visible in Japan and an urgent priority among its doctors. Its sufferers ranged from the moderately well-off to the most elite. Two seventeenth-century shoguns—Tokugawa Iemitsu (r. 1623–1651) and Tokugawa Ietsuna (r. 1651–1680)—were rumored to have suffered from the disease.[32] Katsuki Gyūzan, in a 1699 treatise that was one of the first Japanese books on *kakke*, identified it with what laymen were calling *Edo wazurai*, "the affliction of Edo [present Tokyo]," an illness that beset those who came to the capital for trade or official duty.[33] Many of the doctors writing about *kakke* had also experienced its symptoms themselves. The Kyoto physician Okamoto Shōan wrote in 1812 that in the past he had experienced the abrupt lower leg swelling characteristic of some types of *kakke*, but initially he simply followed his teacher's instructions to make the appropriate drug and didn't investigate the nature of the illness himself. When the problem recurred years later, however, Okamoto took advantage of two seasons of foot pain–induced immobility to study the treatment of *kakke* in the classics, eventually producing two monographs on the topic.[34]

The eighteenth and early nineteenth centuries were a time of great social and economic change in Japan, as cities burgeoned and consumer culture flourished. After rising to power at the beginning of the seventeenth century, the Tokugawa shoguns had managed to suppress dissent and warfare so effectively that the samurai no longer fought, instead becoming urban bureaucrats. Standards of living rose as the range and amounts of goods available to residents of the cities and castle towns increased. For the first time in Japanese history, trade became "a source of conspicuous wealth, a development to which contemporaries were able to attribute most of the country's ills."[35] In a description that could equally apply to the early modern China that we saw in the previous chapter, Penelope Francks describes eighteenth- and early nineteenth-century Japan as

> a society in which communications and market networks were developing and spreading, while the clearly defined status distinctions of earlier times were breaking down, so that, as the potential for social, as well as geographic, mobility grew, goods took on increasing meaning as indicators of status, taste, and sophistication within wider sections of a fluid society.[36]

Not surprisingly, like Chinese observers of late imperial foot qi, Japanese doctors explained the new *kakke* by suggesting that extravagant lifestyles contributed to causing it. In *Essentials of Kakke* (*Kakke kōyō*, 1861), Imamura Ryōan wrote that the reason *kakke* was most prominent in Edo (that is, Tokyo) was that "among the crowds of gentlemen, fish and salt were plentiful and consumer goods are abundant . . . they have too much and there is nothing they can't obtain. This," he concluded, "is concomitant with the geographical features," such as the low, damp terrain that resembled China's Jiangnan, the original home of foot qi. For Imamura, in other words, the environment was a necessary but not a sufficient factor to explain *kakke* incidence. Changing, decadent habits—produced by the transformation of the military samurai into urban gentlemen—were also a part of the story.[37]

Kakke treatises drew on classical Chinese texts about foot qi to explain the new scourge, but they also deployed ideas not seen in that literature. A new group of doctors today considered part of the Current of Ancient Formulas (*kohōha*) had begun to develop in Japan.[38] They focused on the *Treatise on Cold Damage Disorders* (*Shōkanron*), a Chinese text on fevers written around AD 200, and eschewed the abstract doctrines in other medical classics. From the eighteenth century *kohōha* partisans increasingly promoted the idea that all diseases involve poison that needs to be expelled and that a doctor can locate the poison by systematically palpating the abdomen.[39] Many of the explanations for the new *kakke* reflected this group's influence, centering on poison. In *Types of Kakke*, Okamoto Shōan ascribes some types of the disease to water poison inside the body, acquired in one of two possible ways. In the case of royalty and aristocrats, "when they are young they take in the moldy *qi* [pronounced *ki* in Japanese] of their wet nurses," a new form of the old-fashioned *qi* invasion. An ordinary patient, though, more likely contracted the disease because of "a little fetal poison he has not yet managed to vent."[40] Fetal poison was toxic matter left over from gestation that every infant and child was thought to carry, having acquired it either from ingesting impure substances in utero or from the impure sexual heat generated during conception. The idea of fetal poison as a source of disease had emerged in China only a few centuries earlier when smallpox became so endemic that it was a universal childhood experience. Under such circumstances, it seemed that every child's body contained the seeds of the illness, which would inevitably manifest before adulthood. Smallpox, then, was both scourge and purge; a child who survived a serious bout with the disease had safely vented the fetal poison, and it posed no further danger.[41] In Japan, fetal poison came also to be linked with *kakke*; Okamoto Shōan suggests that fetal poison could have effects beyond childhood and beyond smallpox if it were not fully expunged.[42]

Historians usually treat this surge of early modern *kakke* as an epidemic of beriberi, but I think it is wise to be more cautious.[43] It is possible that the gentlemen of Edo and Osaka were suffering from a thiamine deficiency. Francks has shown that, during this period, eating polished rice on its own, rather than mixed in a porridge with other grains as was typical in the countryside, became fashionable in the cities, and rice constituted a much higher proportion of the diets of prosperous Japanese than it had before.[44] Other scholars have traced the origins of modern sushi to early nineteenth-century Edo.[45]

It is conceivable that consuming a lot of thiamine-destroying raw fish (and alcohol, of which there was no shortage) alongside polished rice may have produced vitamin B deficits. On the other hand, the diets of the comfortable classes were unlikely to have been monotonous enough to bring about clinical symptoms of a nutritional deficiency, and the symptoms described are not, as biomedical doctors say, pathognomonic; many other causes produce similar symptoms. They resemble, for example, the signs of contemporaneous foot qi in China or gout in Europe. The *kakke* symptoms that portended death—dementia, heart failure—are like late-stage symptoms of syphilis. Contemporaneous observations that twenty- to forty-year-old men were most vulnerable to the heart symptoms further bolsters the syphilis hypothesis, which Liao Yuqun has articulated.[46] But ultimately the data we have—descriptions of symptoms, unsystematic observations of epidemiology and consumption patterns—are insufficient to sustain a biomedical diagnosis.

Beyond the problem of data, retrospectively assigning a biomedical diagnosis to this premodern epidemic is a kind of presentist hubris, as the introduction to this book has suggested. It imposes later categories—conditioned by later ideas, biases, and anxieties—on what Tokugawa gentlemen were experiencing, making those later categories more important than the ideas, biases, and anxieties that shaped the gentlemen's own understanding. Worries about latent poison, overindulgence, and environmental miasmas are relegated to trivia, whereas concerns about micronutrient levels are made to seem universal.

By the turn of the twentieth century, a new *kakke* had emerged, reflecting a different set of concerns and afflicting a different segment of the population—and this new *kakke* one can indeed identify as beriberi, because doctors and scientists at that time did so. But the beriberi of late nineteenth-century Japan was not the *kakke* of eighteenth-century Japan, whether or not a thiamine deficiency brought about the symptoms of both; *kakke* did not become beriberi until historical actors gave it that name. Let us turn now to the moment when the histories of beriberi and *kakke* converged, and the modern concept of beriberi was created.

National *Kakke* and the Creation of Beriberi in Japan

Starting in the 1870s, *kakke* took on a new meaning in Japan. The patterns that had emerged in the previous century continued, as merchants and "those of sedentary employments" continued to fall ill.[47] But to these sufferers were added much larger numbers of soldiers, sailors, and students—all segments of the population newly subjected to institutional life under the Meiji regime. *Kakke* became a concern of the nation, a national disease, and the government turned for its solution to newly minted experts in Western medicine.

During the last thirty years of the nineteenth century, Japan underwent dramatic political, economic, intellectual, and social change. For the previous two and a half centuries, the Tokugawa shoguns had presided over what has come to be called a "closed country," in which contact between Japanese and Westerners was strictly limited. By the mid-nineteenth century, a number of nations backed by increasingly powerful navies were eager to open Japan to Western trade and settlement, as the first Opium War had recently opened China next door. In the end it was the Americans, seeing in Japan a potential refueling stop for their steamships, who prodded the shogunate to change its isolationist policies. U.S. Commodore Matthew Perry arrived at the capital with four gunships in 1853 and presented a list of demands such as preferential trade arrangements and the right to station in Tokyo a representative of American interests. The shogun, faced with disproportionate military might and with the example of China's unsuccessful resistance to Western imperialism in the Opium War of 1839–1842, reluctantly acceded to Perry's demands.

In the ensuing fifteen years, it looked as though Japan were headed down the same road as China, a path of economic and political decline that was turning a once-proud empire into a hypercolony riven among multiple Western powers. The script turned out quite differently for Japan, however, because in 1868 the shogun was overthrown in a revolution. The revolution's historical name, the Meiji Restoration, is deceptively conservative. Ostensibly it represented a restoration of the power of the emperor, whose executive prerogatives the shogun, a military ruler, had usurped for the previous seven hundred years. In reality, however, the Restoration was nothing like a return to Japan's classical period.

The new leaders of the Japanese government, the oligarchs surrounding the young Meiji emperor, were mostly former midrank samurai and *daimyō* (regional lords) who had had relatively high positions in the old social order but who had not been at its pinnacle and had had little prospect of getting there. They were determined to fend off Western aggression by transforming Japan into a Western-style empire able to win a place of respect among the existing great powers. Accordingly, one of the first decisions the new government made when the dust of the revolution had settled was to send an official mission to Europe and the United States to renegotiate the unequal treaties that had been made over the previous decade and a half and to study the institutions that they believed made Western nations powerful: their militaries, governmental structures, and educational and legal systems. Subsequently, in the 1870s and 1880s, the oligarchs created a national military, a public education system, and a constitution featuring a bicameral legislature, all based on Western models.

They adopted, also, a belief about health that was increasingly common in Western governments: that a nation's power and prospects lay in part in the bodies of its citizens and that the state therefore had the prerogative—indeed, the responsibility—to inspect, protect, and improve those bodies. In 1875 the Meiji government established a bureau of public health that immediately busied itself drawing up regulations to control and dispose of organic filth. As Ruth Rogaski has shown, the term for the bureau's remit, *eisei*, was drawn from classical Chinese, but it carried none of its classical meaning in this new usage.[48] The old *eisei* had meant "guarding life," indicating dietary, meditative, exercise, and sexual practices that an individual could undertake to protect his or her health and live longer; in Meiji officials' use *eisei* meant what Rogaski calls "hygienic modernity." It entailed policing behavior and monitoring the condition of the masses.

When the bureau was established, one of the public health consequences of Meiji Japan's transformation was already becoming very clear. Large-scale *kakke* epidemics began not long after the Restoration. The nucleus of this public health crisis lay in the new conscript army. Built on the Prussian model, the Meiji military was equipped and trained like European services. Meiji sailors traveled on ships bought from Europe, carried European-made arms, and wore Western-style uniforms. They did not, however, eat European rations of wheat biscuit, peas, and salted beef. Unlike the government of the Tokugawa period, which had given its military men food rations plus a modest extra allowance for meat and vegetables, the Meiji government originally paid its troops in cash. Many conscripts ate cheaply to send the remainder of their income home. This meant diets of mostly polished rice—only the destitute would eat brown—and the effect quickly became apparent.[49] The men began to suffer a disease that was by that time foreign to European ships. The symptoms started in the feet and calves and often involved either swelling or painful shrinking and hardening after which the feet and ankles began to curve, rendering the victim too weak to stand or walk. As the disease progressed, the men would sometimes suffer constipation and urinary retention, lose their appetites, and finally succumb in a violent spasm. So pronounced was the problem that *kakke* became the "national disease" of Meiji Japan.[50]

Although the *kakke* label would have made sense to someone familiar with classical Sino-Japanese medicine, as many of the symptoms in historical accounts of *kakke* were similar to those that Japanese soldiers were suffering, this *kakke* afflicted a different population from the recorded *kakke* of days past. What Okamoto and Imamura had grappled with earlier had been the ailment of well-off sedentary people. It continued to exist and to plague the elite: the Meiji emperor himself endured a bout in 1877, and an imperial princess was said to have died of the disease around the same time. The new *kakke*, in contrast, afflicted people low on the social ladder such as conscripts from poor rural families; they died of an illness that never touched their officers. Most *kakke* observations and statistics in the late nineteenth century came from hospitals, many of which were founded to treat the poor and to segregate those with diseases suspected of being infectious (including, at this time, beriberi).[51]

If the distribution of *kakke* epidemics was new, so too was the orientation of the physicians called on to deal with them. *Kakke's* new experts were not, like Okamoto and Imamura before them, *kampō* doctors working from the classical Sino-Japanese medical tradition. Instead, they belonged to a new generation trained in Western medicine. They looked at blood and sputum samples under microscopes. They systematically altered rations and recorded the results in charts. They assessed the chemical composition of various foods in laboratories. They experimented: they measured and tabulated and calculated; they published in international journals and participated in international conferences. This reflected the dramatic rise in Western medicine's status under the new Meiji government. Although elite doctors in both urban and rural Japan were exposed to and curious about Western medicine well before the late nineteenth century, until the Restoration it had had no connection with or support from the government.[52] After the Restoration, the new government viewed Western medicine as an essential element of its modernizing tool kit. The public health bureau issued regulations for medical licensing that compelled doctors to learn Western medicine; it set up hospitals and medical schools. The Meiji government also supported Western medicine by promoting both study abroad and study with the Germans, Dutch, and English working in Japanese hospitals. The new Kakke Hospital, founded in 1878, included practitioners of *kampō* at the emperor's command, but the very form of the endeavor—controlled, hospital-based research—privileged the Western model of knowledge making, and it was Western-style doctors who dominated there.[53] A new law in 1906 officially relegated traditional practitioners to third-class status, after university-trained and medical school–trained practitioners of Western medicine.[54] And when the Diet established a Kakke Research Council in 1908, its members were, to a man, bacteriologists.[55] Post-1868 Japanese doctors were continuously exposed to the theories then current in Western medicine and to the problems that most confounded Western-style doctors.

Takaki Kanehiro (1849–1920), the naval physician whose experimental modifications of rations brought *kakke* rates in the navy down to negligible levels, perhaps best exemplifies this conjunction of a new disease with a new perspective. Though he studied some *kampō* in his youth, Takaki was far better versed in Western medicine than in the Sino-Japanese medical tradition. At age seventeen he began studying with Ryosaku Ishigami, who had been trained in Dutch medicine (*ranpō*) in Nagasaki, and a few years later he became a student of William Wills, an Edinburgh-trained doctor with the British legation. After working for the navy for a few years, Takaki continued his studies in London, at St. Thomas's Hospital Medical School. His performance there was outstanding, and he won several prestigious awards before returning home. His credentials in Western medicine were, in short, impeccable. Furthermore, though he achieved fame as a *kakke* expert, Takaki was not acquainted with the older *kakke* of the wealthy, the one that Japanese physicians had been writing about since Katsuki Gyūzan's day. He writes that 1872, when he first began to treat sailors at the Naval Hospital, was the first time he had seen the disease. He encountered it only in this institutional setting, not in individual well-heeled patients like the ones described in medical literature before 1868.[56] Between 1872 and 1875, Takaki saw hundreds of cases of this disease at the Naval Hospital. "In summer-time," he wrote, "several acute cases used to appear daily. At times, five or six cases had to be treated simultaneously, and house-officers were obliged to work very hard through the day and night."[57] Hard though they worked, however, the doctors saved few of *kakke*'s victims.

By the time Takaki took over the Tokyo Naval Hospital in 1880, having spent the previous five years studying in London, the problem had grown much worse. Over a third of the sailors in the navy contracted *kakke* each year; after cholera, it afflicted more men than any other disease.[58] Takaki despaired at the numbers. "At times, when the disease was in full sway," he reported, "we found the hospital too small, and often had to use neighboring temples [to house patients]." With the military so enfeebled, it seemed as if the fate of the nation were at risk: "The conditions at such times used to strike my heart cold, when I thought of the future of our empire; because if such a state of health continued without the cause and treatment of *kakke* being discovered, our navy would be of no use in time of need."[59]

Takaki, who had absorbed the ideas current among his London mentors about minimally sufficient diet and its necessary components—thought at the time to be just protein, carbohydrates, and fats—suspected the problem might lie in what the men ate. He convinced the navy leadership to stop giving sailors money for food and to distribute rations instead. He then compared the effects of Western rations with those of Japanese provisions. The experimental Western diet, which included bread in place of rice, eliminated kakke almost completely from the units in which it was used. Because some of the men disliked the Western-style rations and refused to eat them, Takaki tried other modifications and finally struck on barley mixed with rice as a salutary and inoffensive addition to the sailors' diet. It proved just as effective. For his innovations, he was eventually made a baron.[60]

Takaki's main critics were not champions of classical Sino-Japanese medicine—who, as we have seen, had lost much of their cultural authority since the Meiji Restoration. Instead, it was his counterparts in the army, Western-trained physicians themselves, who criticized his approach. The factions visible in Western medicine in Japan resembled those in Europe at the time and reflected the Meiji government's choice to send its army and navy physicians to different countries for training.[61] Great Britain, whose navy was then nonpareil, received the naval physicians, whereas their colleagues from the army went to Germany. Consequently, naval physicians like Takaki came home steeped in the epidemiological perspectives that predominated in England, whereas army physicians returned with strong faith in bacteriology, having spent years in the German laboratories at the cutting edge of that emerging discipline. This produced a different scientific culture in the Army Medical Bureau from the one that prevailed in the Navy Medical Bureau. Army surgeon Ishiguro Tadanori (1845–1943) and his colleagues were so convinced that a microbe caused the *kakke* of sailors and soldiers that they pursued it relentlessly in the laboratory, triumphantly (and mistakenly) announcing the discovery of the causative germ in 1885 and again in 1906.[62] They refused to alter the army's official "scientific" ration of polished rice to imitate Takaki's mixed barley-rice ration. Consequently, in the war against China in 1894–1895 and the war against Russia in 1904–1905, Japanese soldiers sustained much heavier losses from *kakke* than from combat. Sailors had extremely low rates of the disease in comparison.[63] It was not until twenty-three years after the navy adopted *kakke*-preventing dietary reform that the army did the same.

The one thing that virtually all late nineteenth-century researchers agreed on was that the *kakke* they were seeing in Japan was the same as the disease called beriberi elsewhere. As early as 1880 articles began to appear in international medical journals that used the terms *kakke* and beriberi interchangeably, with titles such as "The Japanese Kakke (Beri-beri)," "Kakké, or Japanese Beri-beri," and "On Kak'ke (Beriberi)."[64] In 1887, the Japanese *Sei-I-Kwai Medical Journal* published an article in English titled "Beri-beri (Kakké) in the United States."[65] Duane Simmons, a Western physician resident in Japan for decades after its midcentury opening, observed in "Beriberi, or the 'Kakké' of Japan" that "the name kakké has been used by all the foreign physicians who have published any theory on the disease as observed in this country," lamenting that this was "likely to lead to confusion by implying that it is a distinct malady; whereas its identity with beriberi has never really been disputed."[66] A few scattered observers had, in fact, disputed this identity; one maintained that *kakke* "differs from beriberi in one important point, that very exemption of the Caucasians [who supposedly never get it]."[67] But for the most part, the medical literature of the 1880s and 1890s bears out Simmons's claim; whether European, American, or Japanese, virtually all of those writing about *kakke* for an international audience equated it with beriberi.

The most thorough researchers inquired into local medical knowledge about *kakke*, reporting that "it was named and described by Chinese authors long before anything was written about it by the Japanese."[68] But the mention of earlier Sino-Japanese sources was generally used only to establish how long the disease had afflicted East Asia, not to suggest that there was anything worthwhile about traditional Chinese or Japanese doctors' understanding or treatment of it. In Simmons's words, "A number of Japanese physicians have written on the disease, under the name of kakké . . . Their speculations and conclusions . . . though curious, are hardly worthy of a place in a scientific journal."[69] Already in the 1880s, the antiquity of the disease and the stagnation of non-Western medicine were assumed, reflecting a broader perception at the time that both the diseases prevalent in East Asia and East Asian healing practices were unchanging. Western writers at the same time had begun referring to China as the "cradle of smallpox," ravaged from earliest times by the disease and unable to manage it with their antiquated medicine—even though the Chinese had invented inoculation long before Europeans had ever used it.[70] Beriberi, too, was cast back as a timeless consequence of a timeless bad diet.

Some Japanese physicians tried to maintain a place for distinctively Japanese knowledge in the evolving international literature on beriberi. In his English-language article "On Kak'ke (Beriberi)," the naval physician Yasuzumi Saneyoshi acknowledges the equivalence of the two disease names in the title, but in the essay eschews "beriberi" in favor of "kak'ke."[71] Using the Japanese term instead of the one common in English suggests a proprietary aim, as if to emphasize how much of the current knowledge about the disease was Japanese. If Western scientific journals and international conferences were to begin writing about this disease as *kakke*, that would be an implicit recognition of the Japanese role in observing and managing it. Such efforts never gained much purchase outside of Japanese journals, however. In other international medical journals, *kakke* continued to be presented as a regional variant of the term *beriberi*, appearing less and less frequently until, even in English-language journals published in Japan, it was supplanted entirely by *beriberi*.[72]

This history complicates the narrative that beriberi research in this period is a "success story" of Western or scientific medicine, an opportunity "for Asians to reflect on how much of good the West has brought to their shores," as early vitamin researcher Robert R. Williams wrote.[73] It shows, first of all, that Western medicine was not monolithic: factions of researchers, their approaches informed by national identity as much as anything else, disagreed sharply over what constituted scientific evidence. Ironically, the advocates of bacteriology, whose conclusions we now deem to have been incorrect, attacked as unscientific and mired in tradition the researchers focusing on diet. Ishiguro and his allies derided Takaki's dietary reforms as a form of *kampō*.[74] But Takaki, like Ishiguro, was a Western-style physician with a medical degree, and he championed Western-style medical practice. Barley, which he promoted as a *kakke* prophylactic for those who found bread too exotic, had not figured prominently among the drug ingredients used for *kakke* in traditional medical books. His dietary hypothesis—that the protein, carbohydrate, and fat components of the sailors' diets were mismatched—relied strictly on Western notions of nutrition. Takaki and Ishiguro's conflict was over the value of epidemiological versus laboratory research in understanding disease, not over the validity of Western medicine. They were recapitulating contemporary debates among international practitioners of Western medicine, debates unrelated to traditional medicine.[75] Though Ishiguro attempted to tar Takaki with a *kampō* brush, recognizing that traditional medicine enjoyed lower official support and esteem than Western medicine, his association of Takaki with traditional medicine had no substance.

Moreover, in this case the physicians who were the most outspoken devotees of Western scientific medicine not only did not improve the health of the people in their charge but actually exacerbated suffering because they refused to consider other explanations and interventions. Beriberi killed many thousands of Japanese soldiers between 1894 and 1905 because army doctors insisted that the disease reflected poor hygiene and not the nutrient-poor rations they themselves had mandated. This only added to the irony that the Meiji beriberi epidemics had originally been in part a consequence of the way Western nations' ascendance had reordered local economies and foodways. Steam-milling technology introduced by the West had put the white rice that Japanese consumers esteemed within economic reach of a much broader segment of the population than before. Provisioning a conscript army "scientifically" on the Prussian model had imposed on combat troops a regimen that could not sustain them. If we extend our gaze to include the novelty of the epidemics, in addition to the novelty of knowledge about them, then it is difficult to agree with Williams that this story is an "excellent example of the joining of East and West to mutual advantage."[76]

Elite practitioners of scientific medicine in the late nineteenth century used the term *kakke* synonymously with beriberi, and adduced the antiquity of the term *kakke* to show that beriberi epidemics had in fact plagued East Asia for millennia. That they had finally elucidated such epidemics' true cause showed the superiority of their methods and became an exhibit supporting the case that Japan's Westernization had improved life there. But in this case Westernization had degraded health before improving it. And beriberi research produced not only what we see today as a physiological truth—that micronutrients are necessary to survival—but also much that now looks dubious, such as that beriberi is a tropical disease to which Asian bodies are particularly prone or that traditional Asian food customs were primarily to blame for causing it. Those complicating details disappeared, however, and by the second decade of the twentieth century a streamlined, triumphant narrative about *kakke*'s true identity had spread to Japan's new colonies of Taiwan and Korea and to China as well. That is the story we will examine in the next—and last—chapter.

CHAPTER SEVEN

Foot Qi's Multiple Meanings in Modern East Asia

Foot qi has multiple meanings in East Asian nations today. In Japan and South Korea, it means beriberi. Japanese and Korean dictionaries are unambiguous about this; foot qi (pronounced *kakke* in Japanese, *gaggi* in Korean) is a disorder caused by vitamin B1 deficiency, and there is no alternative interpretation. In Taiwan and the People's Republic of China the situation is less clear. Mainland Chinese dictionaries identify foot qi with beriberi, as they do elsewhere in East Asia, but they generally also include a second meaning: Hong Kong foot or *jiao xuan*, a set of symptoms caused by "a kind of fungus, mostly manifesting in the crevices between the toes" as intense itching and sometimes blisters filled with yellow liquid.[1] This is what Americans call athlete's foot, which entails itching toes and cracking, flaking, or peeling skin on the feet, often accompanied by a foul odor. Search for foot qi on the Chinese edition of Wikipedia today, and you'll find yourself at the "disambiguation" page, which informs the reader that the term has two meanings: beriberi or athlete's foot. Ride the buses and subways in any major Chinese city, and you will see advertisements for antifungal salves to treat foot qi.

Some in the past few decades have tried to differentiate between *foot qi* (*jiao qi*) and *foot qi disease* (*jiao qi bing*), assigning the athlete's foot meaning to the former and the beriberi meaning to the latter. And practitioners of the PRC's two major state-supported forms of medicine—Western medicine (biomedicine) and Traditional Chinese

Medicine—seem to have arrived at a rough division of labor when it comes to the two forms of contemporary foot qi. In biomedical journals, research on foot qi is research into beriberi; a recent article in *Contemporary Medicine*, for example, explores the use of CT scanning to diagnose infants who may have Wernicke's encephalopathy, an extreme stage of beriberi.[2] In journals of Traditional Chinese Medicine, research on foot qi is almost invariably about athlete's foot.[3]

Despite these efforts at "disambiguation," confusion abounds. On Chinese message boards, unfortunate athlete's foot sufferers write in

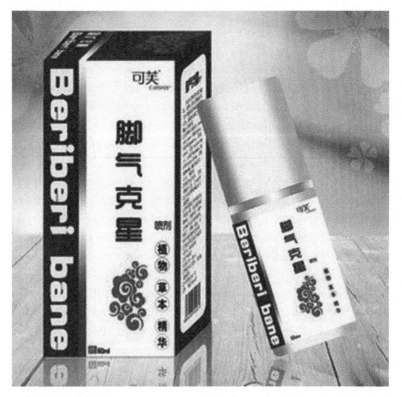

FIGURES 2 AND 3. Topical remedies for the itching, sores, stink, and cracking skin of foot qi (athlete's foot), purporting in English to be "beriberi" treatments.

SOURCES: Beriberi Bane: retrieved on October 8, 2016, from www.jxxesy.com/aspcms/ productlist/list-110-1.html; God Beriberi Oil: retrieved on August 23, 2016, from https:// detail.1688.com/offer/45751661056.html?spm=0.0.0.0.Ai8Ft1.

for suggested remedies and are advised by fellow netizens to take vitamin B supplements.[4] It's easy to see how these well-meaning posters got the idea; websites purporting to be authoritative offer scientific-sounding reasons to explain why vitamin B prevents athlete's foot. One observes that excessive sweat and oil on the feet help cause the condition and then expounds, "Vitamin B can regulate the secretions of the sebaceous glands and increase the skin's strength to resist [infection], thereby helping us prevent the emergence of Hong Kong foot."[5] Conversely, antifungal ointments, sprays, and oils sometimes end up purporting to combat beriberi when the companies that produce them attempt to enhance their products' cachet by translating their names into English, choosing beriberi as the most authoritative translation (Figures 2 and 3).

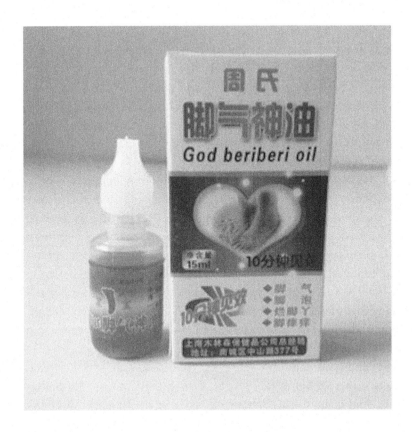

In Taiwan, many have the same perspective on foot qi as people in Japan and South Korea, understanding it as a vitamin deficiency disease. Foot qi appears in historical articles there about Japan's experience with beriberi but not in medical journals. Taiwanese biomedical journals are generally written in English, so the Chinese term's ambiguity does not pose a problem there. The people I spoke with in Taiwan during a visit in 2006, unlike interlocutors in mainland China, assumed immediately when I brought up foot qi that I was talking about beriberi. Still, one sometimes sees foot qi defined as athlete's foot in informal sources such as blogs and message boards based in Taiwan, and as the PRC and Taiwan become more and more economically interdependent, it will likely become more common to see antifungal creams promoted for use against foot qi in Taiwan as well.

In sum, today foot qi's meaning varies by nation and, to some extent, by social or professional groups within a single nation. In Japan and Korea it means beriberi, in the PRC it sometimes means beriberi but more often athlete's foot, and in Taiwan it occasionally means athlete's foot but more often beriberi. This final chapter explores how foot qi acquired its current meanings in mainland China and offers an explanation for why the balance of meanings varies so markedly from one East Asian nation to another. The explanation, as in every previous change we have seen in the meaning of foot qi, is partly epidemiological and partly sociopolitical. Because China industrialized and was integrated into the new global economy later than Japan, the country never experienced a nation-threatening beriberi crisis like its neighbor—that's the epidemiological piece. As for the sociopolitical part: adopting Western medical knowledge, including definitions of disease, became politically important in China by the late 1920s, and consequently physicians adopted the equation between foot qi and beriberi even absent a widespread beriberi problem. But because knowledge about beriberi was more symbolically than practically important, beriberi has proven to be far less durable a disease concept in China than it has been in Japan.

If definitions of disease were solely biological, such diversity would make no sense. Someone must be wrong: the Chinese who understand foot qi as athlete's foot are mistaken, or the Japanese who think *kakke* is beriberi have misunderstood. But definitions of disease are also social and cultural, so it is no surprise that the very different modern experiences of China, Korea, and Japan have left their imprint on modern concepts of disease in those places. Previous research has tended to focus on one national setting only—China but not Korea or Japan, Japan but not Korea or China, Korea but not China or Japan (to say nothing of Vietnam, also part of the East Asian culture sphere).[6] By looking at them together, we can begin to understand the bigger picture: how one shared elite medical tradition, classical East Asian medicine, made room for another—biomedicine—in the modern period. And we can appreciate the variety that persists even within supposedly uniform, hegemonic cultures of knowledge.

Little Beriberi: The Silver Lining to China's Terrible Nineteenth Century

The vitamin B deficiency disease beriberi has never been a major killer in modern China as it was in nineteenth-century Japan. Yes, some unfortunate laborers and migrants suffered from beriberi in the 1920s through 1940s, and refugees struggled with nutritional shortfalls under the Japanese occupation.[7] In the years after the founding of the People's Republic, the terrible famine of the late 1950s induced "water swelling" (starvation edema) among some, to which thiamine deficiency may have contributed.[8] And recent medical journals attest to the occasional appearance of infantile or prenatal beriberi. But beriberi has not figured among the primary health concerns in modern Chinese history. It certainly never became, as it had been in Japan, the "national disease."

When beriberi was ravaging populations in Japan and southeast Asia, Western observers in the 1880s remarked with surprise at how little beriberi there seemed to be in China. Erwin Baelz, observing the *kakke*-beriberi epidemic in Japan, stated that "the Chinese are seldom affected by kakké."[9] Philip Cousland, living in the city of Shantou on the southeast China coast, saw an outbreak of beriberi among students at the missionary school there but noted, "It is very remarkable that I did not hear of a single case in Swatow [Shantou] or the large district of which Swatow is the port."[10] Duane Simmons, writing from Japan, felt that there ought to have been lots of Chinese beriberi and was puzzled that foreign observers had not written about it. Perhaps, he supposed, foreigners resident in China were too sequestered from the native population to have seen it.[11] Perhaps. But the fragmentary evidence that survives suggests that foreign observers were not reporting much beriberi because there was not much beriberi to report.

What data we have about mortality and morbidity in late nineteenth-century China comes from Western missionaries and from foreign officials stationed in treaty ports after the Opium Wars, especially from the Europeans who had taken over China's Customs Service and its income. The most productive source for this kind of information is the *Customs Gazette*, published by the British Inspector General of Customs. From 1871 on, this periodical included a biannual health report from the medical officers stationed in each of the treaty ports. These reports tend to center on the health of the foreign population, as one might expect, but frequent or epidemic disease among the Chinese did not go unnoticed: leprosy, dysentery, and malaria often appear in the *Customs Gazette* as afflictions of the locals. Neither beriberi nor foot qi makes an appearance in them, even in the 1880s and 1890s, when beriberi was most visible abroad. If beriberi had appeared frequently among Chinese patients, one might expect the medical officers to have commented on it in their reports. At the very least, it would have appeared in the mortality and morbidity tables they compiled for their respective hospitals. The annual report of the colonial surgeon in Hong Kong enumerated hospital admissions and deaths in the colony and arranged them by cause. Beriberi does, indeed, appear in these reports, but it is not one of the most prominent causes of admission to the civil hospital. In 1895, for example, out of a total of 2,283 admissions to hospital and 114 deaths, beriberi is listed as the cause of only twenty-two admissions and six deaths. There was only a fraction as many admissions for beriberi as for malarial fever or even gonorrhea.[12] For comparison, a table compiled by Admiral Yasuzumi Saneyoshi of hospital admissions among Japanese soldiers and sailors during the Sino-Japanese War shows beriberi casualties constituting more than half of all illnesses, more than dysentery, malaria, and cholera combined.[13]

The comparative insignificance of beriberi in late nineteenth-century China helps to explain why Chinese physicians writing about foot qi at the time took no notice of the beriberi problem affecting other parts of the world. Most literate Chinese doctors continued to write about foot qi as a complicated disorder with a number of causes and manifestations, to be treated case by case by an experienced doctor. In late nineteenth-century China, even monographs on foot qi did not mention research being done in hospitals and other countries, despite the intensity with which Western-style doctors in other places were scrutinizing beriberi. *Superficial Remarks on Foot Qi (Jiao qi chu yan)*, written by the classical physician Zeng Chaoran in 1887, betrays no inkling about the *kakke* epidemics that had been ravaging the military in Japan, or Takaki's successful treatment of the disease in Japan's navy. For the most part Zeng's book covers old ground, discussing the difference between wet and dry foot qi, the prevalence of the disease in the south, and "immoderate eating and drinking" as its internal cause. There are a few new elements—for example, an observation about how women in Vietnam try to expel foot qi with betel nut—but no influence from contemporary discussions of beriberi.[14]

A second specialist book published nearly twenty years later, Fu Lisheng's *Excellent Tried-and-True Formulas for Foot Qi Syndrome (Jiao qi zheng jing yan liang fang*, 1906) shows even less connection with the beriberi literature of the day. The disease that Fu discusses is one that afflicts "book readers and artisans, people who don't walk or move around much," including, apparently, the author himself. He writes that his lower legs suddenly swelled up after being tender for some months, and he found relief only when a friend who had suffered similar symptoms recommended a fish dish as a remedy. Later on, when friend after friend came down with the same symptoms, Fu passed on the recipe for this anti–foot qi dish to them, each time with good results.[15] The foot qi Fu describes—a chronic, recurring swelling in the lower legs—has more in common with the disorder in sixteenth-century medical books than with early twentieth-century literature on beriberi. Even an author who purports to know about developments in Western medicine, Zhang Hefen, seems oblivious to beriberi and the international efforts to understand it in his 1909 *Summary of the Symptoms of Foot Qi (Jiao qi zheng ji yao)*: "Western doctors," he reports, "say that in this syndrome there is often 'electric poison [*dian du*],' so its manifestation is extremely violent . . . I believe this is so, so you can't use needles [to treat it—that is, acupuncture]. That is, silver needles are also unsuitable to use, lest they conduct the electricity."[16] If Western doctors did, in fact, think such things about foot qi, they do not seem to have written them down.

This highlights another way in which late nineteenth-century China differed from Japan: not only was foot qi less rampant than *kakke*, but also Western medicine was more peripheral. In China, the main source of status was still officialdom and the classics-based civil service exams leading to it.[17] Western medicine had no official support and was introduced almost entirely by foreign missionaries, who worked in China only because the Western powers forced the government to accept them. The relationships between Western and classical East Asian doctors were thus more haphazard and tenuous in China in this period than in Japan, where modernization had been decreed by the state. Close working relations required a certain disregard for social boundaries and expectations. So despite the exhortations of a small number of high-powered proponents of Western science and medicine, traditional practitioners felt little pressure to adopt the priorities and concerns of Western medicine, or even to acknowledge its presence.[18]

The relative absence of beriberi in late nineteenth-century China may have been a thin silver lining to a generally traumatic engagement with Western powers. Like Japan, China had experienced the pressure of demands from industrializing, sea-based Western empires in the mid-nineteenth century. But because China had been so comparatively big and powerful when Western incursions began, the mismatch between Western empires and the Qing empire was neither as great nor as clear as it was between the United States and the Tokugawa shogunate. And, unlike in Japan, where revolutionaries overthrew the shogunate just fifteen years after the start of unequal treaties and encroachment by Western powers, in China the Qing government managed to retain the loyalty of the elite for much longer. The Qing government survived the steady erosion of its legitimacy not only by Western humiliations but also by a devastating civil war for more than half a century. Revolution came only in 1911, after about seventy years of the same depredations that Japan had experienced for fifteen. And unlike Japan, where just a few years after the Restoration the Meiji government was firmly in control and actively transforming the institutions of all of Japan into modern ones, in China the revolution was followed by a decade and a half of chaos as warlords, would-be emperors, and republicans competed to realize their conflicting visions of the nation's future. It was only in 1927, after the Guomindang reunified much of China, that something like a functioning central government emerged. This government was as committed to Western-style modernization and industrialization as the Meiji regime in Japan had been, but they were beginning the process almost sixty years later.

In many ways this late conversion was a disadvantage, as fledgling Chinese industries found it difficult to compete with well-established industry in other countries, but in terms of nutritional deficiency disorders it may actually have been a blessing. None of the factors that had contributed to causing Japan's beriberi epidemics had been present in late nineteenth-century China. The impulse to standardize and Westernize education, medicine, and the military did not hold sway in Qing China as it did in Meiji Japan, despite the "self-strengthening" suggestions of some Chinese reformers. There was no concerted overhaul of the army into a modern-style national military until the Guomindang army started forming in the 1910s. China was not tied in to the emerging economy of global industrialism, except in the treaty ports that Western nations had forced open and in the British colony of Hong Kong—and it was there, indeed, that beriberi appeared, albeit in less dramatic fashion than in Japan.[19] Later, in the 1920s and 1930s, beriberi troubled the Chinese military as well as students and prison inmates but never to the extent that it had afflicted the Japanese. Besides, by then officials understood both the cause of the problem and its solution and insisted that white rice in the regimen of these institutionalized populations be replaced with brown rice and supplemented with beans and barley.[20]

From this perspective, then, China's late conversion to the Western model of development may have been a boon. Crucially, China industrialized only after the understanding of nutritional deficiency disorders had already been worked out. When in 1910 the Far Eastern Association of Tropical Medicine concluded that beriberi was caused by diet, the imperial government was still a year away from crumbling. It took another decade and a half after the 1911 revolution for the new political order to stabilize enough for comprehensive reform of health care to be possible. In other words, by the time China began to industrialize under an effective government, the global beriberi moment had passed.

Beriberi Becomes Foot Qi's Official Chinese Translation

Despite the relative rarity of beriberi in China, the disease became symbolically important to the Chinese elite in the early twentieth century. Like their Meiji counterparts, Chinese leaders in the first few decades of the twentieth century advocated for Western medicine as a matter of self-defense and embraced laboratory medicine and modern nutritional science as emblems of their modernity. Familiarity with the new disease concepts that those sciences had produced became foundational knowledge for responsible citizens. Magazine articles aimed at the new bourgeoisie warned in apocalyptic terms of the beriberi epidemic that would result from eating too much highly refined foreign rice, citing the Japanese experience as precedent.[21]

This change reflected the new prominence of Western science and medicine in China. In the first decade of the twentieth century, the Qing government scrambled to institutionalize Western models to stave off collapse and defend itself against foreign incursions. In 1905 the civil service examinations were abolished in favor of an education system that would emphasize science and technology. Western-style doctors joined their classically trained counterparts in the palace medical service for the first time in 1908. In the coastal cities where the bulk of the population lived, new licensing exams for doctors required familiarity with both Chinese and Western theories and techniques.[22] The imperial family's efforts at reform were not enough to preserve its rule, and after its fall in 1911 students and reformers continued to agitate for scientific and civic development in the maelstrom of political contests among the Guomindang, warlords, and imperial powers. The urgent demands of young Chinese intellectuals, pressing for science and democracy, could no longer be ignored after the May Fourth protests of 1919.

Meanwhile, the direction of knowledge flowing between China and Japan—in the past mostly from the former to the latter—had reversed. Japan became the most important conduit through which recent Western learning entered China. Modern-style schools specializing in science and Western learning proliferated in China, often headed and staffed by Japanese instructors. In a mirror image of seventh-century Japanese delegations that learned medicine in China, in the early twentieth century large numbers of Chinese students headed to Tokyo to study science and medicine.[23] Whether abroad or at Japanese-led schools at home, these students absorbed the knowledge then current in Japan. New coinages poured into their language, crafted by Japanese scholars conversant in both Western science and classical Chinese. Most technical terms in modern Chinese began as Japanese inventions around the turn of the twentieth century. Sometimes the Japanese translators chose novel combinations of characters, as in the two-character compound *kagaku*, created to represent the Western concept of "science." Elsewhere, as we saw in the previous chapter, they assigned new meanings to old compounds, as in the case of *kakke*—foot qi—which became beriberi.[24] Because the concept of foot qi had originally moved from China to Japan back in the sixth through eighth centuries, one might say that the Chinese gave the Japanese a disease, and, by the time the Japanese returned it in the early twentieth century, it was unrecognizable.

By the late 1920s, when the Guomindang finally consolidated power and inaugurated an effective government, Western-style medical practitioners were no longer politically marginal in China. In the last years of Qing rule, future Chinese leaders had seen how imperial powers could use protecting public health as a pretext for violating national sovereignty; they were determined to undermine that rationale for imperial expansion by building a Western-style public health regime themselves.[25] Even the founder of the Guomindang, Sun Yat-sen, had trained as a Western-style medical doctor. So it is no surprise that the officials running the new Ministry of Health were Western-style physicians also, many opposed to classical medicine as backward and detrimental to national development. So confident were these modernizers that in 1929 they passed a resolution at the first National Public Health Conference to abolish traditional medicine altogether. This galvanized practitioners of classical medicine, who began to organize, protest, and court the patronage of the state themselves. Gaining the support of the Guomindang elite, however, required proponents of Chinese medicine to demonstrate that their art too was (or could become) modern and scientific.[26]

For disease concepts, this meant that classical disease names needed to be correlated with scientific entities. What were the *sudden turmoil, flowers of heaven,* and *foot qi* of classical medicine, really? Shi Jinmo, an eminent practitioner of Chinese medicine serving as vice president of the new Institute of National (that is, traditional) Medicine, wrote in 1933 that traditional Chinese disease names, which had "always been incongruent with science," ought to be preserved only in cases where they clearly corresponded to diseases in Western medicine. He argued for "unifying disease names" by subordinating Chinese disease concepts to Western ones.[27] This approach had already materialized in the 1928 updating of a set of government regulations regarding the prevention of infectious diseases. The original regulations, promulgated in 1916, had listed eight diseases to be monitored—eight entities defined by their causative microbes and identical to lists of notifiable diseases that the Japanese government had produced for the home islands and its colony of Taiwan twenty years earlier. What is striking about this list is the Chinese names of the diseases, each of which is followed, in parentheses, by a Latin name written in Roman letters:

1. *hu lie la* (Cholera)
2. *chi li* (Dysentherie)
3. *chang zhi fu si* (Typhus abdominales)
4. *tian ran dou* (Variola)
5. *fa zhen zhi fu si* (Typhus exanthemata)
6. *xing hong re* (Scarlatina)
7. *shi fu di li* (Dyphtherie)
8. *bai si tuo* (Pestis)[28]

Without exception, the Chinese names are neologisms based on Japanese coinages. Most, such as *hu lie la* for cholera, transliterate the sounds in the original Western term. Some, such as *tian ran dou* ("natural pox") for smallpox, attempt to capture the meaning of the Western term. But all imply, as Sean Lei notes, that "individual infectious diseases and their collective category should be marked as radical novelties in the East Asian medical universe."[29]

The updated list from 1928 shows how this assumption of novelty changed. It jettisons most neologisms in favor of classical Chinese disease names: cholera has become *sudden turmoil*, typhus a form of *cold damage*, smallpox *flowers of heaven*.[30] Each classical term has been tethered to a microbe. When Shi Jinmo wrote a few years later that traditional disease nomenclature ought to be subordinated to the disease names of Western medicine, he was thus only affirming on behalf of Chinese medicine an approach that the government had already adopted. Some of Shi's contemporaries held a more nuanced position; the renowned Western-medicine doctor Wu Lien-teh and his colleague Sung Chih-ai examined classical texts on *sudden turmoil* and concluded that most of them "did not and could not describe true cholera. For that dangerous infection, though possibly not entirely absent from old China, was evidently much rarer than, and not so widespread as, in the nineteenth and twentieth centuries." They concluded that "most likely various authors used to assign this name to different more or less well-defined clinical entities among the group of acute gastro-intestinal diseases."[31] When they wrote this in 1933, however, absolutism had already eclipsed such nuance. In official documents, *sudden turmoil* had already become cholera.

Prominent defenders of traditional medicine saw Shi's approach as rank capitulation. They noticed that the initial impetus to create equivalence between Chinese and Western medical terms had come from boosters of Western medicine with no interest in preserving the native tradition: missionaries such as P. B. Cousland, who served as the head of the terminology committee for the China Medical Missionary Association, and vociferous opponents of Chinese medicine such as Tang Erhe and Yu Yunxiu.[32] The influential Xie Guan was one such defender. When he compiled the first-ever dictionary of Chinese-medicine terms in 1921, he abjured scientific redefinitions of old disease concepts and stuck instead to classical citations.[33] He later explained that he thought it inappropriate to use the knowledge and techniques of the present to measure the worth of what doctors in the past had done and understood. Those who "want to use scientific methods to organize [traditional] medical texts," he charged in 1935, "have made no outstanding achievements yet . . . [they are] seeking out and applying the skin and hair of Western medicine [that is, its superficial elements] and destroying the substance and effect of the original philosophy."[34]

The fate of foot qi as a concept bears out Xie's concerns. Because, in its Japanese pronunciation *kakke*, it had already been identified with the thiamine deficiency disorder beriberi, foot qi was an easy term to incorporate into the new scientific nomenclature. Modernizers adopted the translation as a matter of course; the work of defending it had already been done in 1880s Japan. Moreover, the discovery of vitamin deficiency disorders had come to be perceived as one of the signal successes of Western medicine, and the beriberi research that had given birth to the new disease category was accordingly celebrated. Christiaan Eijkman, the Dutch scientist whose research on the diets of beriberi-stricken chickens had hastened the conclusion that something in rice bran prevented it, received the Nobel Prize for this work in 1929. Previous awardees had made breakthroughs in understanding diphtheria, tuberculosis, typhus, malaria, and anaphylaxis; so the recognition of Eijkman and his corecipient Sir Frederick Gowland

Hopkins indicated that vitamin research had joined bacteriology, parasitology, and immunology in the vanguard of Western medicine. Its symbolic significance mandated that would-be modernizers recognize beriberi discoveries as an outstanding achievement, however minor beriberi was as an actual public health concern.

Just as the elucidation of beriberi's cause had become a point of pride for Western medicine, the antiquity of knowledge about foot qi became one for Chinese medicine. The American scholar of materia medica Bernard Read, working in Shanghai in the 1930s and 1940s, tested the ingredients of various classical foot qi formulas and found that some of them did, in fact, contain thiamine and therefore would have helped cure beriberi. He saw this as proof of Chinese medicine's value, and later scholars both Western and Chinese have echoed this conclusion.[35] In their authoritative *History of Chinese Medicine* (1936), Chimin Wong and Lien-teh Wu declared that foot qi had been "the accepted term of beri-beri" in China from the sixth century "to the present time."[36] Joseph Needham and Gwei-djen Lu perceived early mentions of foot qi in Chinese literature as proof of "the antiquity of human knowledge of beri-beri as a deficiency disease."[37] And taking their cue from these reference works and from specialists such as Needham and Lu, other historians have presented foot qi as a thiamine deficiency disorder whenever they have run into the term in primary sources.[38]

Ultimately, however, this effort to elevate Chinese medicine—by crediting it with priority in discovering effective beriberi treatments—actually diminished it. Rather than preserving foot qi as a complex, changing concept in an independent medical tradition, celebrating premodern Chinese intuitions about vitamins turned classical medicine into a footnote to the triumphant story of Western medical progress. However ingenious ancient Chinese remedies for beriberi had been in their time, they were no longer necessary in an age of scientific supplementation and fortification of foods. And their concepts of causation—wind qi, dampness, rich foods—were too quaint to mention. Thus the extensive body of Chinese medical literature on foot qi became, primarily, proof that thiamine deficiency was "a longstanding problem" in China that premodern doctors feebly grappled with.[39] When the foot qi signs they described did not match those of beriberi, the doctors stood accused of "errors in differentiating similar symptoms."[40] Chen Bangxian charged in his 1929 *History of Chinese Medicine* that premodern medical books "confusedly entered arthritis and other symptoms under the general rubric of foot qi."[41] Fan Xingzhun similarly argued that filariasis frequently got mixed up with vitamin B1 deficiency in ancient literature.[42] Japanese historian Yamashita Seizō contended that premodern medical books that recorded symptoms such as "generalized body aches and alternating chills and fever," "sudden redness and swelling in the feet," and "pain in the knees and inability to kneel," were mixing up "rheumatism, arthritis, and gout" with real foot qi.[43] But distinguishing true from false foot qi assumes that modern doctors know more about the disease than did the doctors who diagnosed and treated it, despite the fact that today's data comes from premodern descriptions. A modern scholar cannot meaningfully disagree with Yu Shanren, an eleventh-century doctor who exclaimed, on seeing a patient whose main complaint was a feeling like insects crawling from his foot to his lower back, "This is true foot qi."[44] Doctors' beliefs about disease condition what they observe and what they choose to record, so the patient we see through their texts is the patient they see. In the case of premodern Chinese doctors, this means that the patient is, incontrovertibly, suffering from a Chinese disease and not a biomedical one.

Over time, its definition ceded to Western medicine, classical foot qi has become less and less relevant in Chinese medicine. Understood as beriberi, it contributes little to Chinese medicine's present luster, only conferring a minor claim to past precocity. Accordingly, in the 1980s foot qi disappeared from the textbooks used in colleges of traditional Chinese medicine, and today it is nowhere to be found in the glossaries of traditional Chinese disease terms compiled by two of the world's most authoritative medical organizations, the World Federation of Chinese Medicine Societies and the World Health Organization.[45] The gradual vanishing of classical foot qi from Chinese medicine suggests that, as David Luesink has argued, mundane bureaucratic processes such as drawing up official glossaries did more to diminish classical medicine than did dramatic gestures like the resolution to ban its practice.[46] Now, historical foot qi generally appears as a bit of trivia in a broader narrative about the discovery of nutritional deficiency disorders.

Foot Qi Is Dead; Long Live Foot Qi

This is not the end of the story, though. However determined the governing elite were to reconcile Chinese and Western disease concepts, most Chinese people were not prepared to yield so useful and common a name as foot qi to so narrow and obscure a disease as beriberi. Because there had not been beriberi epidemics in China like the ones that seared themselves into Japanese historical memory, beriberi did not mean much to the average person in early twentieth-century China. Therefore, even as official documents and dictionaries and the glossaries of terminology committees immured the term *foot qi* in the vitamin-deficiency category, people continued to apply it to sores and itching on the skin of the feet and lower legs: athlete's foot.

This was not a new meaning but rather one of the multiple experiences that had historically been included under the foot qi rubric: in late imperial medical documents one finds itchy, scaly feet, sometimes including purulent sores, described as symptoms of foot qi. For example, in *Restoring Vitality in [Cases of] the Myriad Diseases* (*Wan bing hui chun*, 1587), Gong Tingxian describes a case of foot qi in which the soles of the patient's feet itched and radiated heat; when a boiled broth was applied to them, the sores on the feet burst and released liquid.[47] A 1742 edition of Wu Qian's *Yi zong jin jian*, describing "new methods in external medicine," features an illustration of *jiao qi chuang*, foot qi sores, noting that "foot qi sores develop between the knee and the foot on both legs equally; the leg and calf are bloated; yellow liquid comes out of the sores and congeals into yellow scabs." (See Figure 4.) Because it is not on the feet, this is not tinea pedis; and, although the fungus responsible for tinea pedis can infect other parts of the body as well, it doesn't produce fluid-filled sores that burst and crust over. Still, as a skin infection this foot qi is clearly closer to athlete's foot than to any of the biomedical meanings we have seen

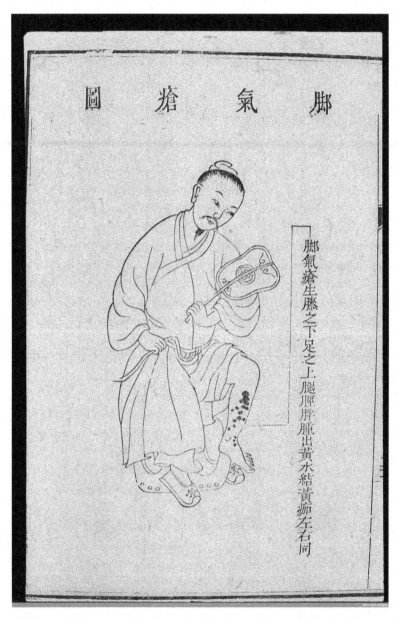

脚氣瘡圖

脚氣瘡生膝之下足之上腿脛胖腫出黃水結黃痂左右同

FIGURE 4. Illustration of foot qi sores, *jiao qi chuang*. Wu Qian, *Yi zong jin jian: Wai ke xin fa*, 1742, juan 71.

associated with foot qi so far and further demonstrates that foot qi as a skin problem is not a recent or inexplicable interpretation. But Western medicine had not decisively conquered athlete's foot as it had beriberi, and compared to the deadly diseases of the early twentieth century a little skin infection was trivial. So although this understanding of foot qi also had a pedigree in historical documents, no one seeking to advance the fortunes of Chinese medicine in the early twentieth century argued that traditional medicine had a noble heritage of treating foot fungus.

In recent years this has begun to change, however. As evidenced by articles on foot qi published in professional journals and the popular press, the persistence of athlete's foot has provided Chinese medicine a new opportunity to compete with biomedicine. Articles on beriberi are rare, confined to occasional pieces on infantile and prenatal beriberi, always in journals of Western medicine or public health.[48] But literature on foot qi as athlete's foot has exploded in the 2000s, perhaps indicating how health concerns have shifted in a newly prosperous China. Utterly overshadowing the rare articles on beriberi are many times as many pieces with titles such as "Why is it so difficult to get rid of foot qi (athlete's foot)?"; here Chinese medicine seems to be holding its own. Popular authors frequently invoke "Chinese medicine's secret athlete's foot remedies," "Folk prescriptions for athlete's foot recommended by Chinese-medicine doctors," and the like. Scientific (or at least, scientistic) papers report the results of experimental trials of Chinese-medicine treatments for athlete's foot.[49] Ironically, having lost authority over foot qi in the early twentieth century by allowing it to become beriberi alone, Chinese medicine is now regaining relevance by laying claim to an alternative meaning that earlier modernizers ignored as too colloquial.

Finally, there are signs that older ways of understanding foot qi are filtering back into discussions among Chinese-medicine practitioners. A recent article in the *Journal of the Liaoning University of Traditional Chinese Medicine* laments:

> Regrettably, when people today bring up foot qi most of them think it is athlete's foot, or only see it as the vitamin B deficiency disorder

of Western medicine, leading the foot qi disease of Chinese medicine to be nearly buried and the discussions of foot qi treatment by medical experts of generations past to be mere ornamentation, with no way to apply them broadly in a clinical setting. This certainly is a shame.[50]

The authors go on to describe the symptoms of foot qi detailed in classical sources, and they conclude that "the gout of modern medicine can be classed in Chinese medicine's 'foot qi disease' category."[51] This represents a new way of looking at classical disease concepts, similar to what this book espouses; the authors do not insist on a one-to-one correlation between Western and Chinese diseases but acknowledge that the latter may correspond to more than one of the former and vice versa. On the ground in China today, then, foot qi continues to be a complex and ambiguous disease concept. Histories of the disease need only catch up.

* * *

China's present foot qi—part vitamin deficiency, part foot fungus, part goutlike pain disorder—reflects a unique constellation of political, economic, and intellectual changes in the modern period. Other East Asian nations changed differently, and consequently their versions of foot qi differ. In Japan, where large numbers of ordinary people suffered from thiamine deficiencies, authorities saw beriberi as a threat to the nation's success, and the embrace of things Western is remembered as a boon, the disease has become equivalent to beriberi. Athlete's foot there is a different term altogether: *mizumushi*, literally "water bug." The Korean case, like the history of Korean medicine more generally, needs more study. The Japanese understanding may well have prevailed in Korea as well, thanks to the enormous intellectual and institutional influence Japan exercised when it governed Korea as a colony between 1910 and the end of World War II. The colonial government put in place something like the tiered system that then existed in Japan, relegating traditional Korean healing (based on classical Chinese medicine) to a second-tier status compared with Western medicine. As Japan made itself model and master, the challenges that the fledgling Japanese nation had faced and overcome in the late nineteenth century became object lessons in Korea, too—and beriberi may have been among them. It may also be the case that as the Japanese appropriated more and more Korean resources for the war effort, including grain, Koreans also had significant experience with nutritional deficiency diseases, and that could have underlined their importance in Korean society.[52] But a clearer picture of how modern Korean disease concepts have evolved awaits further development of a scholarly field just beginning to take shape.[53]

As for Taiwan, it too was a Japanese colony, and many of the dynamics at work in Korea obtained in Taiwan as well. Intending to make Taiwan into a model colony, the Japanese established a public health system modeled on their own and trained Taiwanese nurses and physicians in modern medicine. Moreover, since the Sino-Japanese War fought over Taiwan had also highlighted the Japanese army's beriberi crisis, foot qi-as-beriberi had a special significance in Taiwan's history as well.[54] But the end of the Chinese civil war in the late 1940s sent a second wave of Chinese migrants to Taiwan (the first had been in the seventeenth century), bringing to the island a significant new population with no personal memory of beriberi and with their own persistent understanding of foot qi as athlete's foot. Thus a mix of meanings similar to mainland China's prevails in Taiwan, though the colonial legacy ensures a comparatively prominent place for beriberi within that mix.

And so, in the end, we are left with a contemporary foot qi that highlights the complex dynamics of change in twentieth-century East Asia, just as previous concepts of foot qi did for China and Japan in earlier periods. Just as their predecessors did, educated healers in China today draw on their knowledge and experience to try to relieve what they diagnose as foot qi, whether that be beriberi, athlete's foot, or something else entirely. Just like their premodern counterparts, they are motivated by compassion and by self-interest, informed by their culture and history, and committed to making sense, using the tools and concepts available, of the infinitely variable maladies they encounter. The foot qi that they grapple with, part biochemical process and part social construct, is no more permanent or definitive than its precursors.

What will foot qi become? Single-nutrient deficiencies such as beriberi may continue to recede; gout and arthritis may grow more prominent as Chinese people grow wealthier and live longer; or something entirely different may emerge and come to bear the flexible foot qi name. Hundreds of years hence, historians studying the diseases of China's past may have new scientific concepts to draw on, perhaps some combination of genomics and microbiomics. But to understand what foot qi meant back in the twenty-first century, they will still need to study the social, cultural, and intellectual circumstances that have produced today's disease concepts, just as we have done.

Conclusion

For too long, nineteenth- and twentieth-century translations have been treated like the answer to a question about classical disease concepts in China: "What was that disease, *really?*" In the case of foot qi, "a vitamin B deficiency," the pat answer goes. In contrast, this book has argued that modern translations are more compelling as questions than as answers. Why did beriberi become the official translation of foot qi in the late nineteenth and early twentieth centuries? What does that suggest about how the sources and processing of food were changing in East Asia? About who had epistemological authority? About relationships—between what was becoming Chinese medicine and what was becoming biomedicine; between the governing elite and the common people; among China, Japan, and the West? Seeing the contingency of modern reconceptualizations of Chinese disease—how political, social, and epidemiological circumstances informed them—encourages a more clear-eyed assessment of premodern understandings and more humility about the certainty of present-day knowledge.

The approach that this book has taken to the history of foot qi contributes to current trends in the history of medicine and disease in a few different ways. First, a story like the one you have just read reaffirms that disease is a sociocultural artifact as well as a biological experience, an idea that recent accounts of world-changing diseases have partially obscured. Second, it undermines the impression, widespread today, that Chinese medicine is a monolithic tradition unchanged for several thousand years and that its ideas and practices have always been antithetical to those of Western medicine. And finally, it questions the assumption that the diseases Westerners found in Asia in the late nineteenth and early twentieth centuries were timeless features of life there, miraculously ameliorated by the innovations of Western medicine.

In addition, placing nineteenth- and twentieth-century translations of disease in their historical context can help preserve the relevance of classical medicine and its potential to relieve illness in the future. The epidemiological circumstances of the late nineteenth and early twentieth centuries no longer prevail today. Whereas infectious diseases such as cholera, influenza, and tuberculosis and nutritional deficiencies such as beriberi, pellagra and rickets were the major causes of death and debility a hundred years ago, now noncommunicable diseases such as cancer, stroke, heart disease, and diabetes have taken their place. Even in the poor world, where infectious disease remains prominent, epidemiology is changing; in the early 2000s, the World Health Organization (WHO) reported that the proportion of the global disease burden that noncommunicable diseases represented was about equal, for the first time, to the proportion represented by infectious disease.[1] Cancer is a major and growing problem in Africa, obscured by the attention paid to HIV/AIDS.[2] A classical disease entity whose meaning was sealed in amber in the early twentieth century— as was beriberi, smallpox, or cholera—is likely to be forgotten when beriberi, smallpox, and cholera are no longer significant public health concerns. But, as we have seen in the case of foot qi, the fact that it came to be associated with a disease prominent in the late nineteenth century does not mean that what all Chinese doctors observed about foot qi, and used to treat it, is relevant only to that particular disease.

What premodern Chinese doctors saw and did need not be dismissed as irrelevant in an age of biomedicine, or superseded by biochemistry, as it seemed to have been in the heady decades of mid-twentieth-century medical miracles. Since then, the world has seen the rise of antibiotic-resistant "superbugs"; new infectious diseases such as AIDS, SARS, Ebola, and Zika; and more sophisticated ways of viewing the relationships among microbes and human bodies in the microbiome. These developments have made biomedical understandings of and remedies for infectious diseases seem less complete than they once did, and they have opened the door to renewed examination of what classical Chinese texts have to say. Two examples illustrate this well. The first is the increased interest in traditional Chinese warm-diseases therapies that accompanied the outbreak of SARS in 2003. In mainland China, most SARS sufferers were treated with a combination of Western drugs and Chinese formulas drawn from classical sources on warm diseases (*wen bing*). Outside of China, treatments based on Chinese medicine were largely ignored except as the object of ridicule, but the combined approach would have made sense there, too, given that biomedical remedies were ineffective.[3] More recently, the reexamination of ancient Chinese knowledge about disease has garnered recognition outside of China, in the form of the Nobel Prize awarded to scientist Tu Youyou in 2015 to honor her work in discovering artemisinin, an antimalarial substance. Tu found a reference to the plant from which the drug is derived in a fourth-century text (the text at the center, coincidentally, of Chapter One of this book), which recommended it for use against periodic fevers. By paying close attention to the ancient source's instructions for processing the plant, and by manipulating it experimentally, she and her colleagues produced artemisinin, a providentially effective medicine at a time when drug resistance was beginning to make existing malaria therapies useless.[4]

Such beneficial rediscoveries are only possible, however, if modern understandings of disease names do not obscure their original senses. If the nineteenth-century translation "typhoid" were allowed to stand in for all *cold damage* in the Chinese classics, then the voluminous knowledge about cold damage disorders contained in those texts would seem irrelevant to conditions that are not typhoid, regardless of how similar their symptoms may be. The *nüe* that has been understood as malaria since the early twentieth century was likely also used for intermittent fevers not caused by a plasmodium. But having *nüe* conceptually chained to malaria makes it a less likely place for researchers like Tu Youyou to look for novel ways of dealing with yellow or dengue fever. The problem is even clearer in the case of foot qi. Its diffuse symptoms in the classical sources could, in addition to the beriberi and athlete's foot meanings that it bears today, have reflected heart disease, arthritis, gout, or diabetes. Limited by its modern translations, however, foot qi has sunk into clinical obscurity. It is unlikely that a modern researcher would scour the foot qi literature for ideas about managing any serious medical condition today.

Ironically, proponents and practitioners of Chinese medicine themselves appear poised to cement the hundred-year-old translations of a number of classical disease entities. As Chinese medicine has flourished globally over the past twenty years, a vigorous debate has erupted over whether and how to adopt a standard set of English-language terms to translate the technical vocabulary of Chinese medicine. Although both supporters and opponents of standardization have made compelling arguments, momentum is gathering on the side of the standardizers. A unified nomenclature, they say, is essential to establishing Chinese medicine's professional status and securing official recognition for the practice. The bureaucratic institutions that define modern life—"governmental and regulatory agencies, third-party payers (insurance companies), CAM [Complementary and Alternative Medicine] group practices, hospital administrators"—require uniform terminology to function. Like it or not, we live under the tyranny of diagnosis, and if Chinese medicine wants to survive it must come up with some standard diagnoses.[5] Affirming this bureaucratic imperative, the World Health Organization and the Chinese government have convened committees of practitioners to work on standardizing English-language terminology for Chinese medicine. Independently, the scholar Nigel Wiseman and the doctor Feng Ye produced the magisterial *A Practical Dictionary of Chinese Medicine*, intended to serve as a reference for producing standard translations. A greater degree of uniformity is in the offing, it seems.[6]

Will the new standards preserve the ambiguity and changeability of the original terms? The signs are not promising. Both the WHO committee and the World Federation of Chinese Medicine Societies have proposed disease-name translations that tend to accept the equivalence drawn between Chinese illness terms and the diseases of Western medicine as they are understood today: *sudden turmoil* is "cholera"; *nüe* is "malaria"; *heat sore* (*re chuang*) is "herpes simplex."[7] The PRC committee elaborates that when they say "cholera," they mean cholera in a strictly biomedical sense: "the acute infectious disease caused by infection with the cholera vibrio."[8] To be sure, there are many more names on the list that have not been assimilated to biomedical diseases ("fleshy wilting," "head wind," "running piglet"), but those that have may be doomed to clinical irrelevance, like similar Chinese illness concepts that have already disappeared. Foot qi is among the latter—just as it no longer appears in TCM textbooks in China, it does not feature in the WHO's glossary of Chinese-medicine disease names. Its disappearance speaks volumes: this is no longer a disease we have to worry about, it suggests, so it has no place in contemporary medical practice.

Even scholars who have explicitly opposed privileging biomedical over traditional Chinese concepts have offered translations reinforcing the idea that some Chinese diseases really belong to biomedicine. Nigel Wiseman has criticized biomedical-sounding translations such as *acute conjunctivitis* for *wind-fire eye* (*feng huo yan*) on the grounds that they "[restrict] the validity of the translation to those who understand Western medicine and consider Western medicine to be the greater authority in the definition of disease."[9] To adopt biomedical terms is to translate in a "target-oriented" way, he argues, privileging the frame of reference of the Western audience for whom the sources are being translated to make the Chinese concepts more familiar and acceptable to them. Better to adopt a "source-oriented" approach that prioritizes fidelity to the Chinese original, even if that makes it harder for the audience to read and understand the translation.[10] And yet there are some Chinese terms that even Wiseman is willing to gloss biomedically. In the *Practical Dictionary*, cholera, diphtheria, smallpox, and malaria appear as unproblematic translations of *sudden turmoil, white throat, flowers of heaven,* and *nüe*.[11] Foot qi, though translated as "leg qi," is said to correspond to "beriberi (attributed to vitamin B1 deficiency)" in Western medicine.[12] In sum, when it comes to the diseases that dominated the late nineteenth and early twentieth centuries and defined Western medicine's diagnostic strengths, even Wiseman departs from his generally conservative approach and accepts the biomedical terms as good-enough equivalents for older Chinese ones.

At this moment, then, on the brink of a standardization that will surely elevate some translations and condemn others to disappear, this study recommends taking a view as skeptical of the ones produced around the turn of the twentieth century as of the newer candidates. This would mean extending Wiseman's "source-oriented" principle to include the translations created a hundred or more years ago. Those were no less "target-oriented" than *acute conjunctivitis* is today, after all, devised as they were to make classical medicine legible to determined Westernizers. They prioritized illnesses prevalent at the time but—in most cases—peripheral now. Enshrining them in a bureaucratic apparatus such as the WHO's list of international standard terminologies could limit how attentive practitioners might think to apply the knowledge in Chinese medical classics in the future.[13]

The goal of this book has been to encourage the reader, whether historian, practitioner, or curious soul, to engage imaginatively with East Asian ideas about disease, past and present. Liberated from the belief that understandings of disease have only gotten better and better over time, one can see what is peculiar about modern concepts, how they fit the habitats that the twentieth century created for them. It becomes apparent, for example, that Western imperialism informed modern ideas about disease both by shaping the global disease burden and by making scientific medicine prestigious. We can understand the historical reasons why the same disease name means different things in different parts of East Asia, without misleadingly judging some nations to be less completely modern than others or insufficiently scientific. To appreciate the political, social, and economic factors shaping the biomedical definition of a disease today is not to deny the achievements of modern Western medicine. The discovery that late nineteenth- and early twentieth-century beriberi was caused by vitamin deficits opened up a new, useful way to think about illness and relieved significant suffering in that time. But seeing the political, social, and economic factors makes the limits of those achievements visible. The foot qi that Western-style doctors elucidated and resolved in the early twentieth century was not the foot qi that Chinese physicians faced in the sixteenth century, nor is it the foot qi that troubles many people today. Moreover, although the construction of the vitamin deficiency disease as a category opened up new ways of thinking, it also foreclosed older ways of understanding illness. Gone were the notions that certain body types were more vulnerable; that the same disease in different regions had different causes; that wind and damp sank in through the pores and made one ill; that overeating and drinking too much alcohol impaired the circulation of qi. Excavating those older perspectives has been the major task of this book. If it has induced the reader to take those premodern perspectives seriously, to view them as neither more nor less influenced by political and social context than today's disease concepts, then it has achieved its purpose.

Glossary of Chinese Characters

bai si tuo 百斯脫
bi 痹
bian zheng lun zhi 辨證論治
bing 病
bu fa 補法
chang zhi fu si 腸窒扶斯
chi li 赤痢
chong xin 衝心
chuan xiong 川芎
da wu chen tang 大烏沉湯
da yi jing cheng 大醫精誠
dang gui nian tong tang 當歸拈痛湯
dao yin 導引
eisei 衛生
fa 發
fa dong 發動
fa zhen zhi fu si 發疹窒扶斯
fang feng 防風
fang shu 方書
feng huo yan 風火眼
feng yin tang 風引湯
fu zuo 復作
gan cao 甘草

gong xia pai 攻下派
gu 蠱
hu lie la 虎列剌
huan tui wan 換腿丸
huang qi jian zhong tang 黃芪建中湯
huang qin 黃芩
huo luan 霍亂
jian bu tang 健步湯
jiang qi tang 降氣湯
jiao 腳
jiao qi 腳氣
jiao qi chuang 腳氣瘡
jiao xuan 腳癬
jie 痎
jie yao 節要
jie xi 解溪
jing 精
kampō 漢方
kohōha 古方派
lai 癩
li 癧
lüe yao 略要
ma feng 麻風
ma huang 麻黃
ma ren yuan 麻仁圓
mei du 梅毒
nüe 瘧
qi (ch'i) 氣
qi ren 其人
qing jiao wan 輕腳丸
ranpō 蘭方
re chuang 熱瘡
ren shen 人參
san he san 三和散
shang han 傷寒
shen xian fei bu wan 神仙飛步丸

shi 實
shi fu di li 實扶旳里
tian hua 天花
tian ran dou 天然痘
wen bing 溫病
wu xing 五行
wu yun liu qi 五運六氣
xiao xu ming tang 小續命湯
xie qi 邪氣
xing hong re 猩紅熱
xu 虛
xu ming tang 續命湯
yang sheng 養生
yang yin pai 養陰派
yi 醫
yong quan 湧泉
yuan qi 元氣
yue bi tang 越婢湯
zhang 瘴
zhu fu tang 朮附湯
zhu li tang 竹瀝湯
zi xue 紫雪
zu 足

Notes

Introduction

1. Che Ruoshui, *Jiao qi ji* [Foot qi collectanea].

2. Kanehiro Takaki, "On the Cause and Prevention of Kak'ke" and "Japanese Navy and Army Sanitation."

3. Wang Gang, *Yue liang bei mian*, chapter 2.

4. Examples of historians privileging the beriberi meaning of foot qi include K. Chimin Wong and Wu Lien-teh, *History of Chinese Medicine*, 212; Fan Xingzhun, *Zhong guo bing shi xin yi* [New readings in the history of disease in China], 245; Lu Gwei-djen and Joseph Needham, "A Contribution to the History of Chinese Dietetics," 13; Edward H. Schafer, *The Vermilion Bird*, 133; Yamashita Seizō, *Kakke no rekishi: bitamin hakken yizen.* [History of foot qi: before the discovery of vitamins], 44; Chen Shengkun, *Zhong guo chuan tong yi xue shi* [History of Chinese traditional medicine], 176–181; and Zhang Daqing, *Zhong guo jin dai ji bing she hui shi (1912–1937)* [A social history of diseases in modern China (1912–1937)], 33.

5. *Red Cliff*, DVD, directed by John Woo.

6. Sean Hsiang-lin Lei, *Neither Donkey nor Horse*, 172–177.

7. *Huang Di nei jing su wen: An Annotated Translation*, translated by Paul U. Unschuld and Hermann Tessenow in collaboration with Zheng Jinsheng, 47.

8. Ibid.

9. Sun Simiao, *Bei ji qian jin yao fang* [Essential emergency formulas worth a thousand in gold], 271.

10. Liao Yuqun, "Guan yu Zhong guo gu dai de jiao qi bing ji qi li shi de yan jiu [On the history of foot qi disease in ancient China]." Fu

Youfeng has suggested bubonic plague as the "original meaning" of foot qi, an argument I find unconvincing but that further demonstrates how pliable premodern foot qi is. Fu, "Jiao qi ben yi yu xian shu yi shi hua [Historical discussion of plague and the original meaning of foot qi,]" 25–31.

11. Charles E. Rosenberg, "The Tyranny of Diagnosis."

12. Knud Faber, *Nosography*; and K. Codell Carter, *The Rise of Causal Concepts of Disease.*

13. Andrew Cunningham, "Transforming Plague," 223.

14. In modern Chinese, biomedicine is still referred to as "Western medicine" (*xi yi*), even though it is the predominant form of medicine in China today.

15. Charles E. Rosenberg, "Framing Disease."

16. Steven J. Peitzman, "From Bright's Disease to End-Stage Renal Disease"; and Robert A. Aronowitz, "From the Patient's Angina Pectoris to the Cardiologist's Coronary Heart Disease." Adrian Wilson's "On the History of Disease-Concepts: The Case of Pleurisy" offers another illuminating example.

17. Jeremy Greene, *Prescribing by Numbers.*

18. Andrew Cunningham, "Identifying Disease in the Past."

19. Angela Ki-Che Leung, *Leprosy in China*; and Chia-feng Chang, "Aspects of Smallpox and Its Significance in Chinese History." Leung's "Zhong guo ma feng bing gai nian yan bian de li shi [The history of the evolution of concepts of *ma feng* disease in China]" avoids the problem of casting a modern disease category back onto the ancient concept of *ma feng*, concluding that there's no way of knowing whether *da feng, li/lai,* or historical *ma feng* corresponds to biomedicine's leprosy or not. In contrast, the book *Leprosy in China*, although expressing some of the same uncertainty about the historical identity of *li/lai*, privileges the biomedical understanding by calling the disease "leprosy" in the title.

20. Kerrie L. MacPherson, "Cholera in China, 1820–1930"; and Carol Benedict, *Bubonic Plague in Nineteenth-Century China.*

21. Benjamin A. Elman, *On Their Own Terms.*

22. Marta Hanson, *Speaking of Epidemics in Chinese Medicine.*

23. The originals: William McNeill, *Plagues and Peoples*; and Alfred W. Crosby, *Ecological Imperialism.* Examples of their successors: James L. A. Webb Jr., "Malaria and the Peopling of Early Tropical Africa"; N. D. Cook, *Born to Die*; J. R. McNeill, *Mosquito Empires*; Sheldon Watts, *Epidemics and History*; and George D. Sussman, "Scientists Doing History." Jared

Diamond's best-selling *Guns, Germs and Steel* brought this type of narrative to a more general audience.

24. This tendency among historians to double down on our current understanding of disease rather than interrogating it coincides with what has been called the "neuro-turn" in humanities scholarship, in which scientific discoveries about the brain are used to explain social, psychological, and historical phenomena. This trend has dismayed some historians of science and medicine, who see the neuro-turners as ceding epistemological ground to scientists, undermining the past few decades of scholarship that show how scientific ideas themselves are shaped by culture and by human interests. Roger Cooter, "Neural Veils and the Will to Historical Critique"; and Nikolas Rose, "The Human Sciences in a Biological Age."

25. At least three presses—Johns Hopkins University Press, Oxford University Press, and Greenwood Press—have published "Biographies of Disease" series. Siddhartha Mukherjee's best-selling *The Emperor of All Maladies* employs the same trope.

26. Roger Cooter, "The Life of a Disease?"

27. See Nathan Sivin, *Health Care in Eleventh-Century China*; Bridie Andrews, *The Making of Modern Chinese Medicine*; Sean Hsiang-lin Lei, *Neither Donkey Nor Horse*; TJ Hinrichs and Linda Barnes, eds., *Chinese Medicine and Healing*; Charlotte Furth, "Becoming Alternative?"; Mei Zhan, *Other-Worldly*; Volker Scheid, *Currents of Tradition in Chinese Medicine*; Linda Barnes, *Needles, Herbs, Gods, and Ghosts*; and Volker Scheid, *Chinese Medicine in Contemporary China*.

28. Practitioners of Unani-Tibb ("Greek medicine") in South Asia are the major exception as practitioners who have inherited the ideas and practices of the classical Greco-Islamic tradition and applied them to a different culture, transforming them in the process.

29. Hong Hai lucidly outlines the basic orientations of contemporary traditional Chinese medicine (TCM) in *The Theory of Chinese Medicine: A Modern Explanation*.

30. See, for example, Hong-zhou Wu et al., *Fundamentals of Traditional Chinese Medicine*, 10–13; Hu Dongpei, *Traditional Chinese Medicine*, 3–5; Ted J. Kaptchuk, *The Web That Has No Weaver*, 17–19; and Hong Hai, *The Theory of Chinese Medicine*, 11.

31. Yan Jianhua, "Zhong yi you shi bing zhong zhuan jia diao cha [A survey of experts concerning the types of diseases that Chinese medicine is especially good for]."

32. Angela Hicks, *Discovering Holistic Health*, 14–15.

33. See Volker Scheid, *Chinese Medicine in Contemporary China*; TJ Hinrichs and Linda Barnes, eds., *Chinese Medicine and Healing*, chapters 8–10; James C. Whorton, *Nature Cures*, chapter 11; Joseph S. Alter, *Asian Medicine and Globalization*; and Charlotte Furth, "Becoming Alternative?"

34. Eric I. Karchmer, "Slow Medicine."

35. Yi-Li Wu, "Bodily Knowledge and Western Learning in Late Imperial China."

36. Shigehisa Kuriyama, "Epidemics, Weather and Contagion in Traditional Chinese Medicine."

37. Ted J. Kaptchuk, *The Web That Has No Weaver*, 4. Hong Hai, *The Theory of Chinese Medicine*, 40 and 56, makes a similar claim, saying that Chinese medicine deals with illness or syndromes, not disease.

38. Quoted in Knud Faber, *Nosography*, 70.

39. Volker Scheid, *Chinese Medicine in Contemporary China*, 206.

40. Sean Hsiang-lin Lei, *Neither Donkey Nor Horse*, 172–177; and David Luesink, "State Power, Governmentality, and the (Mis)Remembrance of Chinese Medicine."

41. On sudden and unpredictable change in health policy, see Kim Taylor, *Chinese Medicine in Early Communist China*.

42. Volker Scheid, *Chinese Medicine in Contemporary China*, 212; and Eric I. Karchmer, "Chinese Medicine in Action."

43. Bernard E. Read, *Famine Foods Listed in the Chiu Huang Pen Ts'ao*.

44. A number of observers have cast the mid-twentieth century as the "golden age" of biomedicine, particularly in the United States. For example, Naomi Rogers, *Polio Wars*; John C. Burnham, "American Medicine's Golden Age"; and James LeFanu, *The Rise and Fall of Modern Medicine*.

45. Eric Karchmer, personal communication. Historians and anthropologists of Chinese medicine use the term Traditional Chinese Medicine (TCM), with initial letters capitalized, to label the form of medicine created in the PRC in the 1950s under government auspices and to distinguish it from "traditional Chinese medicine" or "classical Chinese medicine," which could refer to what was practiced before the 1950s or what is practiced outside of China today. Among the distinctive features of TCM are its nationwide standardization through textbooks, examinations, and colleges and the influence of biomedicine on its transmission and practice. See Elisabeth Hsu, *The Transmission of Chinese Medicine*, and Kim Taylor, *Chinese Medicine in Early Communist China*.

46. Bridie Andrews, *The Making of Modern Chinese Medicine*; Sean Hsiang-lin Lei, *Neither Donkey nor Horse*; Volker Scheid, *Currents of Tradition in Chinese Medicine*; and Nathan Sivin, *Traditional Medicine in Contemporary China*, 173–177.

47. The 1933 graph by Pang Jinzhou showing the many varieties of healers and their relationships with one another, reproduced in Sean Hsiang-lin Lei, *Neither Donkey nor Horse*, 122, illustrates this beautifully.

48. Bridie Andrews, *The Making of Modern Chinese Medicine*, 7–8.

49. Sean Hsiang-lin Lei, *Neither Donkey nor Horse*, Introduction.

50. Philip Curtin, *Disease and Empire*.

51. Rudyard Kipling, "The White Man's Burden."

52. William H. McNeill, *Plagues and Peoples*; and Alfred W. Crosby, *Ecological Imperialism*.

53. Jared Diamond, *Guns, Germs and Steel*.

54. David S. Jones, "Virgin Soils Revisited."

55. Christian McMillen, *Discovering Tuberculosis*.

56. Randall Packard, *The Making of a Tropical Disease*.

57. Nancy Stepan, *Eradication*, chapter 2.

58. Roy Porter, *The Greatest Benefit to Mankind*, 465.

59. Richard D. Semba, *The Vitamin A Story*, 151.

60. Kenneth J. Carpenter, *Beriberi, White Rice, and Vitamin B*.

61. For example, Semba notes in passing that the incidence of keratomalacia and xerophthalmia in the Dutch East Indies reached a peak in 1928–1935 that coincided with a threefold increase in imports of sweetened condensed milk from Nestle, the Anglo-Swiss company. This was cheaper than fresh milk, so people who had a little money but not very much started to buy sweetened condensed milk as soon as they were able, with bad public health results (*The Vitamin A Story*, 153–155). But he does not allow this evidence to disrupt the overall picture in the book of triumphant Western discoveries curing a disease endemic to Asia and Africa.

62. David Arnold, ed., *Imperial Medicine and Indigenous Societies*; Roy MacLeod and Milton Lewis, eds., *Disease, Medicine, and Empire*; and Bridie Andrews and Mary Sutphen, eds., *Medicine and Colonial Identity*.

Chapter One

1. Ge Hong, *Zhou hou bei ji fang*, 265. I assume here, based on the work of Chinese philologists, that the foot qi part of the book is original to Ge and not a later addition. Philologists say that it is impossible to tell which parts of *Emergency Formulas* were written by Ge and which came

from the brush of Tao Hongjing, who edited and supplemented the text ca. 500. See Wei Zixiao and Nie Lifang, *Zhongyi Zhongyao shi*, 138. Although Wei and Nie's caution is important, it is reasonable to suppose that the section on foot qi did, indeed, appear in the earliest version. Sun Simiao offers some evidence: he wrote about a large-scale foot qi outbreak among the displaced gentry of the Western Jin after they moved to the area around the capital of the Eastern Jin during the Yongjia reign (AD 307–312). The new capital, Jianye, was about 30 kilometers from Ge's hometown just east of present-day Nanjing.

2. Peng Wei, "Jiao qi bing, xing bing, tian hua," 59–66, 58.

3. H. T. Huang, *Science and Civilisation in China: Fermentations and Food Science*, 582–584.

4. *Huang Di nei jing su wen*, trans. Paul U. Unschuld and Hermann Tessenow, 11. See also David Joseph Keegan, "The 'Huang-ti-nei-ching.'"

5. A number of treatises devoted specifically to foot qi were apparently produced around the same time, but none survives today. We know of their existence because, although the treatises themselves have disappeared, their titles survive in the bibliographies of dynastic histories, which inventory the contents of the imperial library in different periods.

6. Valerie Hansen, *The Open Empire*, 3–6. Another term for this period is the Six Dynasties, recognizing six states as most important. That appellation, however, also privileges dynastic history and obscures some of the most important changes occurring during these centuries.

7. Wan Guodong, "Ge Hong yu *Zhou hou bei ji fang*," 4; and Wei Zixiao and Nie Lifang, *Zhongyi Zhongyao shi*, 136.

8. The most detailed studies of Ge Hong in English are Wells's *To Die and Not Decay*; Campany's *To Live as Long as Heaven and Earth*; Sailey, *The Master Who Embraces Simplicity*; and Ware, *Alchemy, Medicine, Religion*. Outside of medical historians, few scholars cite *Emergency Formulas* or even mention it as a part of Ge's bibliography. Stephen Bokenkamp has even suggested that *Emergency Formulas* was one of the apocryphal texts attributed to Ge Hong after his lifetime: Bokenkamp, "Ko Hung," 481–482 (Ko Hung is an alternative Romanization for the Chinese characters of Ge Hong's name). Medical historians have found no reason to doubt its attribution, however.

9. On the history of the formulary genre, see Ma Jixing, *Zhong yi wen xian xue*, 160. Robert Ford Campany prefers "book of methods" as a translation for *fang shu*, and this makes sense because they describe not only

drug formulas but also physical techniques such as moxibustion (*To Live as Long as Heaven and Earth*, 14).

10. Ge Hong, *Zhou hou bei ji fang*, 196.

11. This suggests that it may have been in common use by his time, a supposition borne out by the presence of specialty treatises on foot qi that were collected in the imperial libraries. Few categories of disorder received such treatment in this period.

12. *Ch'i* is how the character is written in the old Wade-Giles form of romanization; *qi* is how it's written in the now-standard Hanyu Pinyin.

13. Nathan Sivin, *Traditional Medicine in Contemporary China*, 47.

14. Manfred Porkert, *The Theoretical Foundations of Chinese Medicine*; Paul U. Unschuld, *Medicine in China*, 72; and Bridie Andrews, *The Making of Modern Chinese Medicine*, 6, 207.

15. Manfred Porkert coined "heteropathy" as a translation for *xie* to emphasize that the illness-causing *xie qi* differs from the *qi* of the body, invading from the outside. It differs from the *qi* of ingested food, drink, and air because the body is unable to assimilate it. See *The Theoretical Foundations of Chinese Medicine*, 54.

16. Shigehisa Kuriyama, "Epidemics, Weather, and Contagion," 16.

17. Chao Yuanfang, "Zhu bing yuan hou lun," 783–785 (corneal opacity and cataracts), 847 (throat sores), 867 and 870 (cinnabar poisoning), 1002 (wet and dry *jie*, scabieslike symptoms).

18. Zhang Gang, *Zhong yi bai bing ming yuan kao*, 456–464.

19. Ted J. Kaptchuk, *The Web That Has No Weaver*, 4; and Hong Hai, *The Theory of Chinese Medicine*, 40 and 56.

20. Ge Hong, *Zhou hou bei ji fang*, 265.

21. Charles E. Rosenberg, "The Tyranny of Diagnosis."

22. "Lingnan" literally means "south of the mountains," and "Jiangdong" means "east of the river," with "mountains" referring to the mountain range bordering modern Guangxi and Guangdong provinces on the north and "river" referring to the Yangzi River. So Jiangdong and Lingnan are, respectively, the area south of the Yangzi River between Wuhu and Nanjing and the area that is now the provinces of Guangdong and Guangxi.

23. Stephen R. Bokenkamp, "Ko Hung," 481.

24. Sun Simiao, *Bei ji qian jin yao fang*, 265.

25. Edward H. Schafer, *The Vermilion Bird*. The climate of north China may not have been as dry and desolate in the fourth century as it is today.

Paleoclimatological and historical data suggest that it was wetter in the past than it is now. Recent scholarship has also highlighted how much average temperatures in this area have fluctuated over time; see Mark Elvin's *The Retreat of the Elephants*, 3–5, 44, 49; E. N. Anderson's *Food and Environment in Early and Medieval China*, 50–51; and Jonathan Karam Skaff's *Sui-Tang China and Its Turko-Mongol Neighbors*, 28. No one has suggested, however, that the north resembled the south, even then. Certainly the ancient and medieval Chinese elite perceived them differently.

26. Bin Yang, "The Zhang on Chinese Southern Frontiers."

27. *Huang di nei jing su wen*, 332–341.

28. See Keiji Yamada, *The Origins of Acupuncture, Moxibustion, and Decoction*; and Vivienne Lo, ed., *Medieval Chinese Medicine*, 227–251.

29. Though in the past scholars have sometimes translated *wu xing* as "five elements" or "five agents," "five phases," now standard, conveys the Chinese meaning most accurately. The phases are not elements because they describe function rather than composition or structure, so a substance that is water at one time will later become wood as circumstances change. Likewise, they are not agents because the phases merely describe the state of *qi*, which brings about change. For a more extended discussion, see Nathan Sivin, *Traditional Medicine in Contemporary China*, 70–80.

30. Meng Shen, *Shi liao ben cao*, 10.

31. Ibid., 11.

32. David R. Knechtges, "Gradually Entering the Realm of Delight," 236–237.

33. In a pinch, he indicates, goat's milk will also do. Ge Hong, *Zhou hou bei ji fang*, 265.

34. Ibid., 80.

35. Ibid.

36. Vivienne Lo has observed this in her reading of manuscripts and artifacts from early and medieval tombs. In *Medieval Chinese Medicine*, 227–251.

37. The translation here is Shigehisa Kuriyama's, from "Epidemics, Weather, and Contagion," 15n29.

Chapter Two

1. Sun Simiao, *Bei ji qian jin yao fang*, 271.

2. Ibid., 271–272.

3. *Huang di nei jing su wen*, v.1, 326.

4. C. Pierce Salguero suggests using the term *religio-medical marketplace* for this period in China to erode the anachronistic distinction we moderns make between religion and medicine. People in seventh-century China did not perceive these as separate realms. *Translating Buddhist Medicine in Medieval China*.

5. H. T. Huang, *Science and Civilisation in China*, 581.

6. Liao Yuqun, "Guan yu Zhong guo gu dai de jiao qi bing"; and Fan Xingzhun, *Zhong guo bing shi xin yi*, Chapter 5.

7. It is possible that *jing* and *liang*, which together mean "polished rice," are meant to be read separately here, as *jing*—*japonica* rice—and *liang*—foxtail millet. But "polished rice" as an interpretation for *jingliang* is attested in the *Liang History* (*Liang shu*), completed AD 635, so it is also possible that this is the usage Sun intended in his book of the 650s. Sun Simiao, *Bei ji qian jin yao fang*, 271.

8. Robert Somers, "The Sui Legacy," 199.

9. Arthur F. Wright, *The Sui Dynasty*, 7–8.

10. Fabrizio Pregadio, "Chao Yuanfang."

11. Okanishi Tamehito, *Song yi qian yi ji kao* [Studies of medical books of the Song dynasty and earlier], 574.

12. Chao Yuanfang, *Zhu bing yuan hou lun*, 415.

13. Shigehisa Kuriyama has argued that pulse diagnosis was *the* central diagnostic technique in early learned medicine. Although classical Chinese physicians enshrined four techniques as the pillars of diagnosis—asking, looking, listening/smelling (*wen*), and palpating the pulse—they produced specialty monographs on only one: pulse palpation. Shigehisa Kuriyama, *The Expressiveness of the Body and the Divergence of Greek and Chinese Medicine*, 19–20. See also Elisabeth Hsu, "Tactility and the Body in Early Chinese Medicine."

14. Hughes Evans, "Losing Touch."

15. Mu Peng, "The Doctor's Body." This emphasis on experiential, embodied knowledge persists to some extent in modern Traditional Chinese Medicine (TCM). TCM textbooks usually specify fifteen to twenty different descriptors for the qualities of pulses practitioners can expect to encounter in everyday practice. The textbook edited by the Guangdong Province Academy of Chinese Medicine, *Zhong yi lin chuang xin bian*, describes fourteen pulses commonly seen in sick people (60–61), whereas the one on diagnosis and treatment edited by the Shanghai Academy of Traditional Chinese Medicine describes seventeen (82–83).

16. Chao Yuanfang, *Zhu bing yuan hou lun*, 415.

17. For summaries of the ingredients and methods of preparation for versions of Continuing-Life Decoction (*xu ming tang*), Maidservant from Yue Decoction (*yue bi tang*), Bamboo Sap Decoction (*zhu li tang*), and Wind-Drawing Decoction (*feng yin tang*) in formularies that were roughly contemporaneous with *Sources and Symptoms*, see Li Jingwei, Deng Tietao et al., eds., *Zhong yi da ci dian*, 307, 544, 1458–1459, 1466. See also Dan Bensky and Randall Barolet, eds., *Chinese Herbal Medicine*, 89, 397; and Dan Bensky, Steven Clavey, and Erich Stöger, eds., *Chinese Herbal Medicine*.

18. The *yang sheng* tradition is long, predating the systematization of theory in the earliest medical classics, as Vivienne Lo has shown in "The Influence of Yangsheng Culture on Early Chinese Medical Theory."

19. *Huang Di nei jing su wen*, 57.

20. Shigehisa Kuriyama, "Wind and Self," in *The Expressiveness of the Body and the Divergence of Greek and Chinese Medicine*.

21. Livia Kohn, *Chinese Healing Exercises*, 11. See also Livia Kohn and Yoshinobu Sakade, *Taoist Meditation and Longevity Techniques*, chapter 8.

22. "Healing exercises" works well as a translation for *dao yin* in *Sources and Symptoms* because healing is the main object of the text. In some other texts, however, *dao yin* exercises are promoted as a way to extend life or prevent illness; therefore, "longevity and healing exercises" might be a better general translation for *dao yin*.

23. Chao Yuanfang, *Zhu bing yuan hou lun*, 418.

24. Li Jingwei, Deng Tietao et al., eds., *Zhong yi da ci dian*, 1316, 1624.

25. Nathan Sivin, *Chinese Alchemy*, offers both a biography of Sun and a study of his alchemical treatise.

26. Sun asserts, for example, that a great doctor must not consider whether the patient is "high-born or lowly; rich or poor; old or young; beautiful or ugly; enemy, relative, or good friend, Chinese or foreign; stupid or wise"—they must all be treated with the same care.

27. Sabine Wilms, "The Female Body in Medieval China"; and Charlotte Furth, *A Flourishing Yin*.

28. The important *Treatise on Cold Damage Disorders* (*Shang han lun*) is the exception, but Sun apparently got his hands on the *Treatise* after finishing his *Essential Formulas* and used it to complete his *Extended Formulas Worth a Thousand in Gold* some thirty years later.

29. Sun Simiao, *Bei ji qian jin yao fang*, 270.

30. Nathan Sivin, *Health Care in Eleventh-Century China*, 5. Michel Strickmann, *Chinese Magical Medicine* shows in more detail what religious forms of healing consisted of.

31. Fan Ka-Wai, "The Period of Division and the Tang Period," 83.

32. Nathan Sivin, "Text and Experience in Classical Chinese Medicine."

33. The reconsolidation of power probably affected patronage in a way similar to what happened after the consolidation of one of the first bureaucratic dynasties, the Han, back in the third century BC. Geoffrey Lloyd and Nathan Sivin have written about the bureaucratization of expertise attending this previous consolidation of authority in *The Way and the Word*, 28–42.

34. Vivienne Lo, "The Han Period," 40.

35. Sun Simiao, *Bei ji qian jin yao fang*, 266.

36. Chao Yuanfang, *Zhu bing yuan hou lun*, 413-414.

37. Some editions read "one to three months" instead of "one to three days"; editor Ding Guangdi suggests that somewhere along the line of transmission, "day" was mistranscribed as "month," an easy mistake to make as the Chinese characters for these words are very similar. Chao Yuanfang, *Zhu bing yuan hou lun*, 414–415.

38. Sun Simiao, *Bei ji qian jin yao fang*, 271.

39. Quoted in Tamba no Yasuyori, *Ishimpō*, 183.

40. Sun Simiao, *Bei ji qian jin yao fang*, 271.

41. Chao Yuanfang, *Zhu bing yuan hou lun*, 29–30.

42. Sun Simiao, *Bei ji qian jin yao fang*, 267.

43. Ibid., 268.

44. Chao Yuanfang, *Zhu bing yuan hou lun*, 416.

45. The "mountain passes" Sun refers to are those around the border between modern Henan and Shaanxi provinces, in north-central China. Sun Simiao, *Bei ji qian jin yao fang*, 266.

46. Shigehisa Kuriyama, "Epidemics, Weather, and Contagion."

47. Confucius, *The Analects*, Book XII, section 19; Book II, sections 1 and 3. We know today, of course, that the apparent rotation of other stars around the North Star is an illusion, but observers in the time of the *Analects*, ca. 4th century BC, did not know this.

48. Mencius, *The Works of Mencius*, 201.

49. Fabrizio Pregadio, *Great Clarity*, 76.

50. E. N. Anderson, *Food and Environment in Early and Medieval China*, 3, 174–175.

51. Chao Yuanfang, *Zhu bing yuan hou lun*, 29–30.

52. Sun Simiao, *Bei ji qian jin yao fang*, 270.

53. Ibid., 269.

54. Shigehisa Kuriyama, "Blood and Life" in *The Expressiveness of the Body*.

55. Roel Sterckx, "Food and Philosophy in Early China," in Roel Sterckx, ed., *Of Tripod and Palate*. See also John Kieschnick, "Buddhist vegetarianism in China," in the same volume.

56. Fan Ka-Wai, "*Jiao Qi* Disease in Medieval China," 1001.

57. Liao Yuqun, "Guan yu Zhong guo gu dai de jiao qi bing"; and Fan Xingzhun, *Zhong guo bing shi xin yi*.

58. H. T. Huang, *Science and Civilisation in China*, 581.

Chapter Three

1. *San li* was a point on the body's circulation tracts, located a few inches below the knee.

2. Zhang Congzheng, *Ru men shi qin*, 27.

3. Ibid.

4. See Dan Bensky, Steven Clavey, and Erich Stöger, eds., *Chinese Herbal Medicine*, 634–638, 673–680.

5. That is, aching or numbness, or weakness that makes it difficult to bend or extend the limbs. *Bi*, the term Zhang uses here, is a term that does appear in the *Yellow Emperor's Inner Canon*, unlike foot qi.

6. Zhang Congzheng, *Ru men shi qin*, 29.

7. Even Zhang's implication that a legitimate disorder is one that appears in the *Inner Canon* reflects the contribution of the Song government. In large part it was the Song government's issuing of standard editions of selected medical classics that created something like a medical canon for the first time. Accordingly, earlier doctors writing about foot qi had not cared that the term did not appear in the *Inner Canon*. In the seventh century, Su Jing acknowledged neutrally that "from ancient times there was no name foot qi," and explained that "people of later generations" adopted the name based on the observations that swelling and bloating starting in the lower legs often characterized these disorders. Su Jing, preserved in Wang Tao, *Wai tai mi yao fang* [Arcane essentials from the imperial library], 336.

8. On Song activism in education, Thomas H. C. Lee, "Sung Schools and Education"; on the economy, Paul J. Smith, "State Power and Eco-

nomic Activism during the New Policies," and Cecilia Lee-fang Chien's introduction to *Salt and State*; and, in daily life, Patricia Ebrey, "The Response of the Sung State to Popular Funeral Practices," and Peter K. Bol, "Government, Society and State."

9. Patricia Ebrey and Maggie Bickford, eds., *Emperor Huizong and Late Northern Song China*; and Asaf Goldschmidt, *The Evolution of Chinese Medicine* and "Huizong's Impact on Medicine and Public Health."

10. TJ Hinrichs, "Governance through Medical Texts and the Role of Print."

11. Officials had occasionally been instructed to provide drugs for epidemic relief in earlier dynasties, but the Song marked the first time that this became a routine function of government. See TJ Hinrichs, "Governance through Medical Texts and the Role of Print." Song officials also worked to curtail responses to disease that they considered medically undesirable and immoral, such as avoiding contact with sick relatives: TJ Hinrichs, "The Medical Transforming of Governance and Southern Customs."

12. Asaf Goldschmidt, "Commercializing Medicine or Benefiting the People?"

13. Ibid. See also TJ Hinrichs, "The Song and Jin Periods."

14. TJ Hinrichs, "Governance through Medical Texts and the Role of Print," 218–219. As Hinrichs also notes, the number of official medical texts that the Northern Song government produced was much greater than the number that subsequent governments produced, as well: thirty-three official medical texts in 166 years of the Northern Song, versus fourteen over the course of the following 240 years. See TJ Hinrichs, "The Medical Transforming of Governance," 113.

15. Liao Yuqun et al., *Zhong guo ke xue ji shu shi, yi xue juan*, 299.

16. Ibid.

17. The *hui min* and *heji ju* in the title of this work refer to two different elements of the state system for producing and providing drugs. *Hui min ju* (Benefit the People Bureau) was the name of the shops that sold the preprocessed drug formulas, whereas a *he ji ju* (Harmonizing Prescriptions Bureau) was responsible for preparing the drug ingredients and ensuring quality control. Liao Yuqun et al., *Zhong guo ke xue ji shu shi*, 302–304. For the sake of simplicity, I have chosen to translate the two components with the single title "imperial pharmacy" because both were parts of the same drug-provision system.

18. These are all formulas recommended for foot qi in the official formularies of the Song: Gold Sprouts Wine, *jin ya jiu*; Banksia Rose Pills, *mu xiang yuan*; Noble Dendrobium Powder, *shi hu san*; Rhinoceros Horn Decoction, *xi jiao tang*. Most of these are not listed in Dan Bensky and Randall Barolet, eds., *Chinese Herbal Medicine: Formulas & Strategies*, but see 76–77, 273, 457–458.

19. Liao Yuqun, Fu Fang, and Zheng Jinsheng, *Zhongguo kexue jishu shi*, chapter 4.

20. Joseph P. McDermott, *A Social History of the Chinese Book*.

21. Tsuen-Hsuin Tsien, *Science and Civilisation in China*, 146–172.

22. Liao Yuqun et al., *Zhong guo ke xue ji shu shi, yi xue juan*, 299.

23. It is not clear when exactly *Easy, Concise Formulas* was written, but textual exegeses have dated it between 1190 and 1220. Yuan Bing, "*Song dai fang ji xue cheng jiu yu te dian yan jiu*," 74–75.

24. Wang Shuo, *Yi jian fang* [Easy, Concise Formulas].

25. Liu Chenweng, *Xu xi ji*, 469b.

26. Among the critical responses were Lu Zuchang's *Supplementary Treatise on* Easy, Concise Formulas (*Xu yi jian fang lun*), Shi Fa's book of the same title, and (most famously) Zhu Zhenheng's *Beyond the Imperial Pharmacy Formulary* (*Ju fang fa hui*). See Fan Xingzhun, *Zhong guo yi xue shi lue*, 122–123.

27. Wang Huaiyin, *Tai ping sheng hui fang*, 1368.

28. Ibid., 1385; and Shen Fu et al., *Zheng he sheng ji zong lu*.

29. Wang Huaiyin, *Tai ping sheng hui fang*, 1368.

30. Scholars generally capitalize the names of organ systems in classical Chinese medicine to emphasize that Chinese physicians perceived organs as functional systems and cared little about them as physical objects. For an opposing view, however, see Yi-Li Wu, *Reproducing Women*, chapter 3.

31. Nathan Sivin, *Traditional Medicine in Contemporary China*, 124–133, 213–236.

32. Ge Hong, *Zhou hou bei ji fang*, 265.

33. Charlotte Furth discusses the emergence of women's medicine as a field in this period in *A Flourishing Yin*.

34. Chao Yuanfang, *Zhu bing yuan hou lun*, 415.

35. Chen Cheng et al., *Tai ping hui min he ji ju fang*, 308. The formulas mentioned are *huang qi jian zhong tang, xiao xu ming tang, zhu fu tang, zi xue, san he san, ma ren yuan, jiang qi tang*, and *da wu chen tang*. See Dan

Bensky and Randall Barolet, eds. *Chinese Herbal Medicine,* 224, 396, 229, 419.

36. Zhu Zhenheng, one of the "four famous doctors of Jin and Yuan," criticized the formulary directly in his writings; others, such as Zhang Congzheng, attacked it more obliquely.

37. Asaf Goldschmidt, "Commercializing Medicine or Benefiting the People."

38. Zhang Congzheng, *Ru men shi qin,* 28.

39. Wang Huaiyin, *Tai ping sheng hui fang,* 1368.

40. World Health Organization, "History of the Development of the ICD."

41. Angela Leung, "Organized Medicine in Ming-Qing China."

Chapter Four

1. Wang Huaiyin, *Tai ping sheng hui fang,* 1355.

2. Dong Ji, *Jiao qi zhi fa zong yao,* 419a.

3. For example, H. T. Huang, *Science and Civilisation in China,* 578–586; Liao Yuqun, "Guan yu Zhong guo gu dai de jiao qi bing"; and Angela Ki Che Leung, "Japanese Medical Texts in Chinese on Kakké."

4. Chen Bangxian, *Zhong guo yi xue shi,* 342.

5. The others were Liu Wansu (1110–1200), Zhang Congzheng (1156–1228), and Zhu Zhenheng (1281–1358).

6. Li Gao, as quoted in Dong Su, *Qi xiao liang fang,* 298. The books referred to in the quotation are *Emergency Formulas Worth a Thousand in Gold (Beiji qian jin yao fang)* of AD 652, *Arcane Essentials of the Imperial Library (Wai tai mi yao)* of AD 752, and the *Medical Encyclopedia: A Sagely Benefaction of the Regnant Harmony Era (Zheng he sheng ji zong lu)* of AD 1117, all of which have been mentioned in earlier chapters.

7. Li Gao, as quoted in Dong Su, *Qi xiao liang fang,* 298.

8. As quoted in Zhu Su, *Pu ji fang* (Universal aid formulary), 3875.

9. Yu Tuan, *Xin bian yi xue zheng chuan,* 386.

10. Herbert Franke and Denis Twitchett, eds., *Alien Regimes and Border States.* See also Thomas J. Barfield, *The Perilous Frontier,* chapters 5 and 6; and Hoyt Cleveland Tillman and Stephen H. West, eds., *China under Jurchen Rule.*

11. Morris Rossabi, *China among Equals.*

12. Catherine Despeux, "The System of the Five Circulatory Phases and the Six Seasonal Influences." Today phase energetics is usually not included

in the curricula of modern schools of Chinese medicine, and some Chinese historians tend to discuss it with an almost embarrassed air. Typical is Fan Xingzhun, *Zhong guo yi xue shi lue*, 134, in which he says that phase energetics "constituted an obstacle to medical development."

13. It sounds much better in the rhyming Chinese: *bu du wu yun liu qi, bian jian fang shu he ji.* Fan Xingzhun, *Zhong guo yi xue shi lue*, 133.

14. Zeng Shirong, *Huo you kou yi*, 41.

15. *Huang di nei jing su wen*, 332–341.

16. Li Dong-yuan, *Treatise on the Spleen and Stomach*, 8.

17. Ibid., 24.

18. Zhang Canjia, *Zhong yi gu ji wen xian xue*, 127.

19. Qiu Peiran, *Zhong guo yi ji da ci dian*, entry I0005, 758.

20. What I translate as *primordial qi* (following Nathan Sivin, *Traditional Medicine in Contemporary China*, 238, 261) is a term that seems to appear much more frequently in the late imperial texts than in their predecessors. The term (and variant versions such as *yuan qi* and *zhen qi*) appears in the ancient medical classics. Late imperial disease literature often discusses the danger of damaging or depleting it.

21. Li Gao, *Yi xue fa ming*, 553b–554a.

22. Sun Simiao, *Bei ji qian jin yao fang*, 271.

23. As quoted in Wang Tao, *Wai tai mi yao fang*, 340.

24. Li Gao, *Yi xue fa ming*, 553b–554a.

25. Ibid.

26. Zhu Su, *Pu ji fang*, 3875.

Chapter Five

1. Dai Yuanli, *Tui qiu shi yi*, 20.

2. Ibid.

3. Ibid.

4. Liao Yuqun, "Guan yu Zhong guo gu dai de jiao qi bing"; Fan Ka-Wai, "*Jiao Qi* Disease in Medieval China"; Angela Ki-Che Leung, "Japanese Medical Texts in Chinese on Kakké," 164; H. T. Huang, *Science and Civilisation in China*, 578–586; and Gwei-djen Lu and Joseph Needham, "A Contribution to the History of Chinese Dietetics."

5. Evelyn Rawski, "Economic and Social Foundations of Late Imperial Culture"; Michael Marmé, *Suzhou*; and Craig Clunas, *Superfluous Things*.

6. Benjamin A. Elman, *A Cultural History of Civil Examinations in Late Imperial China*, 251–252.

7. Timothy Brook, *The Confusions of Pleasure*.

8. Lucille Chia, *Printing for Profit*; and Tsuen-Hsuin Tsien, *Science and Civilisation in China*.

9. Christopher Cullen, "*Yi'an* (Case Statements)."

10. Li Shizhen, *Ben cao gang mu*, vol. 1, 194.

11. Joanna Grant, *A Chinese Physician*, chapter 4.

12. Sun Simiao, *Bei ji qian jin yao fang*, 272.

13. Su Jing's book on foot qi was lost long ago, but fragments survive in Tamba no Yasuyori. *Ishimpō* [Formulas at the heart of medicine], 182.

14. Ibid,, 183.

15. Physicians used some drug formulas to induce sweating, believing that when a sickness was still superficial the pernicious *qi* could thus be forced out through the skin.

16. Ibid., 183. It is unclear what Gold Sprouts refers to here. Purple Snow is a compound drug consisting mostly of minerals and costly ingredients such as flakes of rhino horn, mentioned among other places in Li Shizhen's *Systematic Materia Medica*, vol. 1, 646. The costliness of such a remedy, meant to be kept at hand as an everyday therapy, contributes to the impression that premodern foot *qi* sufferers were an affluent lot.

17. Yu Tuan, *Xin bian yi xue zheng chuan*, 386.

18. In present-day Shaanxi Province, not far from Xi'an.

19. Jiang Guan, *Ming yi lei an* [Categorized case records of famous doctors], 178b, 180b, 178b.

20. Dai Yuanli, *Mi chuan zheng zhi yao jue ji lei fang* [Secretly, orally transmitted methods for diagnosis and treatment], 54.

21. Li Chan, *Yi xue ru men* [Introduction to the study of medicine], 521.

22. Zhang Shiche, *Ji jiu liang fang* [Excellent formulas for rescuing people in emergency aituations], 676.

23. Angela Ki Che Leung, "Japanese Medical Texts in Chinese on *Kakké*."

24. Yu Tuan, *Xin bian yi xue zheng chuan*, 388.

25. Zhu Su, *Pu ji fang*, vol. 4, 3929.

26. Gong Tingxian, *Wan bing hui chun*, 10–11.

27. Jiang Guan, *Ming yi lei an*, 178a, 179b, 180b.

28. Zhu Su, *Pu ji fang*, 3875.

29. Jiang Guan, *Ming yi lei an*, 179a, 180b, 181a.

30. Victor W. Rodwell, *Harper's Illustrated Biochemistry*. *Harper's Biochemistry* is commonly used in American medical schools today to teach basic physiology and pathology.

31. Lou Ying, *Yi xue gang mu*, 318.

32. Zhang Jiebin, *Jing Yue quan shu*, 701.

33. Li Yongcui, *Zheng zhi hui bu*, 304.

34. As quoted in Marta Hanson, "Northern Purgatives, Southern Restoratives," 153.

35. Ibid. This was almost certainly true, considering that Xue was one of the highest-ranked medical officials in the empire.

36. Angela Ki Che Leung, "Medical Instruction and Popularization in Ming–Qing China"; Chao Yüan-ling, *Medicine and Society in Late Imperial China*, Chapter 4; Robert Hymes, "Not Quite Gentlemen?"; and Benjamin Elman, *A Cultural History of Civil Examinations*.

37. Wang Kentang, *Zheng zhi zhun sheng*, 248b.

Chapter Six

1. Norio Shimazono and Eisuke Katsura, *Review of Japanese Literature on Beriberi and Thiamine*; and Robert R. Williams, *Toward the Conquest of Beriberi*, chapters 4 and 7.

2. Kenneth J. Carpenter, *Beriberi, White Rice, and Vitamin B*; Robert R. Williams, *Toward the Conquest of Beriberi*; and George W. Bruyn and Charles M. Poser, *The History of Tropical Neurology*, chapter 1. Accounts of other nutritional-deficiency disorders are similarly triumphant, for example Richard D. Semba, *The Vitamin A Story;* Francis E. Cuppage, *James Cook and the Conquest of Scurvy*; Stephen R. Bown, *Scurvy*; and Kenneth J. Carpenter, *The History of Scurvy and Vitamin C*.

3. Judith A. Bennett, "Germs or Rations?" For a contrasting perspective, see K. Codell Carter, "The Germ Theory, Beriberi, and the Deficiency Theory of Disease."

4. "The Far Eastern Association of Tropical Medicine."

5. Rima D. Apple, *Vitamania*. For more on the cultural effects of the vitamin revolution in the West, see Gyorgy Scrinis, *Nutritionism*; Harvey Levenstein, *Revolution at the Table*; and Harmke Kamminga and Andrew Cunningham, eds., *The Science and Culture of Nutrition*.

6. Kenneth J. Carpenter, *Beriberi, White Rice, and Vitamin B*, 204.

7. Ibid., xi.

8. William McNeill, *Plagues and Peoples*, chapter 1; and Thomas McKeown, *The Role of Medicine*, chapter 4.

9. William Johnston, *The Modern Epidemic*.

10. Yamashita Seizō, *Kakke no rekishi*, 24–25; and B. Scheube, *Die Krankheiten der Warmen Länder*, 208.

11. Edward Vedder, *Beriberi*, vii. The Scottish Orientalist Sir Henry Yule, who compiled a dictionary of Anglo-Indian terms in the late 1800s, was likewise cautious about the origins of *beriberi*. Henry Yule, *Hobson-Jobson*, 87.

12. Ibid., 88.

13. John Grant Malcolmson, *A Practical Essay on the History and Treatment of Beriberi*, 5n.3.

14. On the Dutch, see Kenneth Carpenter, *Beriberi, White Rice, and Vitamin B*, 12. On the American experience, see Robert Williams, *Toward the Conquest of Beriberi*. On beriberi among sugarcane workers, see Judith Bennett, "Germs or Rations?" On beriberi in Japan, see Alexander R. Bay, *Beriberi in Modern Japan*.

15. Quoted in Kenneth Carpenter, *Beriberi, White Rice, and Vitamin B*, 7.

16. Eduard Jeanselme, "Le Béribéri," 121. Translation my own.

17. David Arnold, "British India and the 'Beriberi Problem,'" 307–308.

18. Larissa N. Heinrich, *The Afterlife of Images*, 256. See also Mark Harrison, *Climates and Constitutions*, 11–14, on how essentialized understandings of race began to change concepts of disease in the late nineteenth century.

19. "The Far Eastern Association of Tropical Medicine," 1229.

20. Michael Worboys, "The Discovery of Colonial Malnutrition," 222.

21. The 1855 date for the advent of steam-milled rice is given by George Bruyn and Charles Poser in *The History of Tropical Neurology*, 6.

22. Ken DeBevoise, *Agents of Apocalypse*, chapter 5.

23. Roy Porter, *Greatest Benefit to Mankind*, chapter 15; and Michael Shiyung Liu, *Prescribing Colonization*, chapter 1.

24. See Patrick Manson, *Tropical Diseases*.

25. Randall Packard, *The Making of a Tropical Disease*; J. M. Powell, *Bring out Your Dead*; Stephanie Haensch et al., "Distinct Clones of *Yersinia pestis* Caused the Black Death"; and William C. Summers, *The Great Manchurian Plague*.

26. Harrison, *Disease and the Modern World*, 133–138; Randall Packard, *The Making of a Tropical Disease*; Roy Porter, *The Greatest Benefit to Mankind*, 462–492; and David Arnold, ed., *Imperial Medicine and Indigenous Societies*, Introduction.

27. Masayoshi Sugimoto and David L. Swain, *Science and Culture in Traditional Japan*; and Margaret Lock, *East Asian Medicine in Urban Japan*, chapter 4.

28. Li Jingwei and Lin Zhaogeng, *Zhong guo yi xue tong shi, gu dai juan*, 212.

29. Andrew Edmund Goble, *Confluences of Medicine in Medieval Japan*; and John Z. Bowers, *Medical Education in Japan*.

30. In these texts *kakke* is apparently discussed as a consequence of injuries sustained in battle. See Andrew Edmund Goble, *Confluences of Medicine in Medieval Japan*, 97.

31. Liao Yuqun counts twenty-eight such books in the *History of Diseases in Japan in the Meiji and Earlier*. Liao Yuqun, "Ji zai yu quan shi."

32. Ibid.

33. Alexander R. Bay, *Beriberi in Modern Japan*, 15.

34. Okamoto Shōan, *Kakke bunrui hen*, 1.

35. W. G. Beasley, *The Meiji Restoration*, 42.

36. Penelope Francks, "Inconspicuous Consumption," 144. Ironically, considering the similarities with contemporaneous foot qi in China, Japanese doctors associated new *kakke* with the foot qi of early Chinese texts only, arguing that the Chinese literature after the eleventh century was about something other than the kind of *kakke* they were seeing. Japanese doctors emphasized the dangerous heart-attacking symptoms of the disease, the fatal spasm, over the less lethal symptoms of chronic leg pain and swelling. And they thought of medieval China as a peaceful and prosperous society like their own. See Angela Ki Che Leung, "Japanese Medical Texts in Chinese on Kakké."

37. Imamura Ryōan, *Kakke kōyō*, preface.

38. I follow Volker Scheid in translating *ha* (Chinese *pai*) as "current." Volker Scheid, *Currents of Tradition in Chinese Medicine*, 11–13.

39. Margaret Lock, *East Asian Medicine in Urban Japan*, 53–55; and Yasuo Otsuka, "Chinese Traditional Medicine in Japan."

40. Okamoto Shōan, *Kakke bunrui hen*.

41. Charlotte Furth, *A Flourishing Yin*, 178–182; and Chia-feng Chang, "Aspects of Smallpox," 54–66.

42. Okamoto Shōan, *Kakke bunrui hen*.

43. Yamashita Seizō, *Kakke no rekishi*; Alexander R. Bay, *Beriberi in Modern Japan*, 11; Christian Oberländer, "The Rise of Scientific Medicine

in Japan," 177–180; and Penelope Francks, "Inconspicuous Consumption," 144.

44. Penelope Francks, "Simple Pleasures," 101–106. See also Emiko Ohnuki-Tierney, *Rice as Self*, 15.

45. Jordan Sand, "How Tokyo Invented Sushi."

46. Liao Yuqun suggests syphilis in "Ji zai yu quan shi," 121–154. Takao Suzuki, *Palaeopathological and Palaeoepidemiological Study of Osseous Syphilis in Skulls of the Edo Period* implies an incredibly high syphilis rate of 54.5 percent among Tokyo residents in the seventeenth to nineteenth centuries. Curiously, however, Ann Bowman Jannetta does not mention syphilis in *Epidemics and Mortality in Early Modern Japan*.

47. Duane B. Simmons, "Beriberi, or the 'Kakké' of Japan," 44.

48. Ruth Rogaski, *Hygienic Modernity*, 151.

49. Liao Yuqun, "Maifan nanjue."

50. Albert S. Ashmead, "Some Observations on Kakké"; Alexander R. Bay, *Beriberi in Modern Japan*, chapter 3; and Kenneth J. Carpenter, *Beriberi, White Rice, and Vitamin B*, chapter 1.

51. Susan L. Burns, "Contemplating Places," 705–709.

52. Ellen Gardner Nakamura, *Practical Pursuits*; H. Beukers et al., *Red-Hair Medicine*; and John Z. Bowers, *Western Medical Pioneers in Feudal Japan* and *When the Twain Meet*.

53. Alexander R. Bay, *Beriberi in Modern Japan*, 32–35.

54. As early as 1875, getting a license to practice medicine in Japan required that one pass an examination in *Western* medicine. John Z. Bowers, *Medical Education in Japan*, 37.

55. Alexander R. Bay, *Beriberi in Modern Japan*, 88.

56. Kanehiro Takaki, "Japanese Navy and Army Sanitation," 421. Takaki's biographical information comes from Liao Yuqun, "Mai fan nan jue"; Yoshinori Itokawa, "Kanehiro Takaki"; and James R. Bartholomew, *The Formation of Science in Japan*, 57.

57. Kanehiro Takaki, "Japanese Navy and Army Sanitation," 421.

58. Ibid. Itokawa gives a figure of 4,327 illnesses per 1,000 soldiers but does not reveal where his data comes from. Yoshinori Itokawa, "Kanehiro Takaki (1849–1920)," 538.

59. Kanehiro Takaki, "Japanese Navy and Army Sanitation," 422. There may also have been beriberi epidemics among the Japanese population at large at this time, similar to what happened in the Philippines, but little research has demonstrated the prevalence of beriberi outside of the military

in nineteenth-century Japan. A few doctors at the time suggested that many civilians were also being admitted to hospitals with a diagnosis of *kakke*, but a more definite conclusion about civilian beriberi awaits a closer inspection of primary sources by a specialist in Japanese history.

60. Liao Yuqun, "Maifan nanjue"; and Kenneth J. Carpenter, *Beriberi, White Rice, and Vitamin B*, chapter 1.

61. Roberto Padilla, "Science, Nurses, Physicians and Disease," 70.

62. Ibid., 83, 104.

63. Alexander R. Bay, *Beriberi in Modern Japan*, 45–50, 64–72.

64. B. Scheube, "Die Japanische Kak-ke (Beri-beri)"; and Y. Saneyoshi, "On Kak'ke (Beriberi)."

65. "Beri-Beri (Kakké) in the United States."

66. Duane B. Simmons, "Beriberi, or the 'Kakké' of Japan," 39.

67. Albert S. Ashmead, "Some Observations on Kakké," 168.

68. Ibid.

69. Duane B. Simmons, "Beriberi, or the 'Kakké' of Japan," 41.

70. Heinrich, "How China Became the 'Cradle of Smallpox.'"

71. Y. Saneyoshi, "On Kak'ke (Beriberi)."

72. For example, Sakae Oseki, "Beriberi Like Disease in Mammalian Animals"; and Kenta Ohomori, "Studies on the Cause and Treatment of Beri-Beri in Japan."

73. Robert R. Williams, *Toward the Conquest of Beriberi*, viii.

74. Ishiguro Tadanori, *Kakke ron*, 1b; and Liao Yuqun, "Mai fan nan jue," 45–48.

75. For useful analyses of the debates on clinical versus laboratory knowledge, see Harry Marks, *The Progress of Experiment*, chapter 1; John Harley Warner, *The Therapeutic Perspective* and *Against the Spirit of System*; and Bruno Latour, *The Pasteurization of France*. On the state of nutritional science at the time, see Harmke Kamminga and Andrew Cunningham, eds., *The Science and Culture of Nutrition*; and Elmer Verner McCollum, *A History of Nutrition*.

76. Robert R. Williams, *Toward the Conquest of Beriberi*, viii.

Chapter Seven

1. Luo Zhufeng, chief ed. *Han yu da ci dian*, 6:1278.

2. Yan Jinghui, "Ying you er nao xing jiao qi bing CT zhen duan fen xi ji jian bie zhen duan."

3. As one example: Ding Xiaolin and Tan Hongjun, "Jiao qi yao wu de yan jiu gai kuang."

4. "Jiao qi bing zen me zhi liao? [How do you treat foot qi disease?]," Baidu Zhidao.

5. "Yun fu you jiao qi qian wan bie luan yong yao [Pregnant foot qi sufferers must not recklessly use medicine]," 39 Yu'er Pindao. http://baby.39.net/a/140927/4481265.html.

6. Among the outstanding studies that stay within the boundaries of modern nations: for China, Bridie Andrews, *The Making of Modern Chinese Medicine* and "Tailoring Tradition"; and Sean Hsiang-lin Lei, *Neither Donkey Nor Horse*; for Japan, Ellen Gardner Nakamura, *Practical Pursuits*; and Morris Low, *Building a Modern Japan*; for Korea, Soyoung Suh, "Korean Medicine between the Local and the Universal: 1600–1945"; and for Vietnam, C. Michele Thompson, *Vietnamese Traditional Medicine*. Studies that have begun to create a larger regional understanding include Ruth Rogaski, *Hygienic Modernity*; and Michael Shiyung Liu, *Prescribing Colonization*. Charlotte Furth and Angela Ki Che Leung, eds., *Health and Hygiene in Chinese East Asia* includes articles that focus on Taiwan, Hong Kong, and mainland China but does not explicitly integrate them or approach them comparatively.

7. Hou Xiangchuan et al., *Nutritional Studies in Shanghai*. But Liao Yuqun compiles hospital admissions data showing that foot qi was not a major illness in the 1930s, even in rice-subsisting regions: "Guan yu Zhong guo gu dai de jiao qi bing," 210.

8. Rae Yang, *Spider Eaters*, 61.

9. As quoted in Albert S. Ashmead, "Some Observations on Kakké," 168.

10. Philip B. Cousland, "Notes on the Occurrence of Beri-Beri or Kakké at Swatow," 54.

11. Duane B. Simmons, "Beriberi, or the 'Kakké' of Japan," 40.

12. "Hong Kong Acting Colonial Surgeon's Report for 1895." Carol Benedict displays the information from the colonial surgeons' reports in tables in *Bubonic Plague in Nineteenth-Century China*, Appendix B, 181, 185.

13. Chart reproduced in Ruth Rogaski, *Hygienic Modernity*, 158.

14. Zeng Chaoran, *Jiao qi chu yan*. On internal causes, 9b. On prevalence in the south, 11a–b. On women in Vietnam, 12a–b.

15. Fu Lisheng, *Jiao qi zheng jing yan liang fang*, 9a-10a.

16. Zhang Hefen, *Jiao qi zheng ji yao*, 2b.

17. Benjamin Elman, *A Cultural History of Civil Examinations in Late Imperial China*.

18. David Wright, *Translating Science* and "The Translation of Modern Western Science in Nineteenth-Century China."

19. Robert R. Williams, *Toward the Conquest of Beriberi*, 11–12.

20. Seung-Joon Lee, "The Patriot's Scientific Diet," 1821–1822; and Zhang Daqing, *Zhong guo jin dai ji bing she hui shi (1912–1937)* [A social history of diseases in modern China], 33–34.

21. Seung-joon Lee, *Gourmets in the Land of Famine*, 166–168.

22. Bridie Andrews, *The Making of Modern Chinese Medicine*, 112–144.

23. Robert R. Williams, *Toward the Conquest of Beriberi*, 11–12.

24. Michael Lackner, Iwo Amelung, and Joachim Kurtz, eds., *New Terms for New Ideas*.

25. Ruth Rogaski, *Hygienic Modernity*, chapter 6; and William Summers, *The Great Manchurian Plague of 1910–1911*.

26. Sean Hsiang-lin Lei, *Neither Donkey nor Horse*; and Bridie Andrews, *The Making of Modern Chinese Medicine*, "Tailoring Tradition," and "Tuberculosis and the Assimilation of Germ Theory in China."

27. As quoted in Sean Hsiang-lin Lei, *Neither Donkey nor Horse*, 173.

28. Zhang Zaitong and Xian Rijin, eds., *Min guo yi yao wei sheng fa gui xuan bian* [Selected laws and regulations from the Republic of China regarding medicine and public health], 10.

29. Sean Hsiang-lin Lei, *Neither Donkey nor Horse*, 169.

30. Zhang Zaitong and Xian Rijin, eds., *Min guo yi yao wei sheng fa gui xuan bian* [Selected laws and regulations from the Republic of China regarding medicine and public health], 48.

31. Lien-teh Wu and Sung Chih-ai, "Huo-luan," 16.

32. P. B. Cousland, "Medical Nomenclature in China"; Zhang Daqing, "Gao si lan [Cousland]"; and David Luesink, "State Power, Governmentality, and the (Mis)Remembrance of Chinese Medicine," 164.

33. Xie Guan, *Zhong yi da ci dian* [Great dictionary of Chinese medicine], 3595–3599.

34. Xie Guan, *Zhong guo yi xue yuan liu lun* [On the origins of Chinese medicine], 56a, 57a–b.

35. Bernard E. Read, *Famine Foods Listed in the Chiu Huang Pen Ts'ao*; and Lu Gwei-djen and Joseph Needham, "A Contribution to the History of Chinese Dietetics," 19.

36. K. Chimin Wong and Wu Lien-teh, *History of Chinese Medicine*, 212.

37. Lu Gwei-djen and Joseph Needham, "A Contribution to the History of Chinese Dietetics," 13.

38. See Edward H. Schafer, *The Vermilion Bird*, 133, for an especially exuberant example.

39. *Encyclopedia Britannica* (available at www.britannica.com/science/beriberi) asserts that "in East Asian countries, where polished white rice is a dietary staple, beriberi has been a long-standing problem."

40. Yamashita Seizō, *Kakke no rekishi*, 44.

41. Chen Bangxian, *Zhong guo yi xue shi*, 342.

42. Fan Xingzhun, *Zhong guo bing shi xin yi*, 245.

43. Yamashita Seizō, *Kakke no rekishi*, 44.

44. Jiang Guan, *Ming yi lei an*, 178b.

45. Li Zhen-ji, ed. *International Standard Chinese-English Basic Nomenclature of Chinese Medicine*, 381–403; and World Health Organization, *WHO International Standard Terminologies on Traditional Medicine in the Western Pacific Region*, 162–177. On the disappearance of foot qi from TCM textbooks in the 1980s: Eric Karchmer, personal communication. Interestingly, the Chinese government's Committee to Examine and Approve Chinese Medicine and Pharmacy Terminology does include foot qi in its glossary, translating it "weak foot." Zhong yi yao xue ming ci shen ding wei yuan hui [Committee to examine and approve Chinese medicine and pharmacy terminology], *Zhong yi yao xue ming ci* [Chinese terms in Traditional Chinese Medicine and pharmacy], 252.

46. David Luesink, "State Power, Governmentality, and the (Mis)Remembrance of Chinese Medicine."

47. Gong Tingxian, *Wan bing hui chun*, 318.

48. For example, Tu Ya et al., "Ying er nao xing jiao qi bing 6 li wu zhen bao dao [A report on 6 cases of misdiagnosed neurological beriberi in infants]."

49. For example, Hu Ling, "Lao Zhong yi tui jian de zhi liao jiao qi pian fang [Folk prescriptions for treating foot qi (athlete's foot), recommended by senior Chinese-medicine doctors]"; and Zhang Shuhua et al., "Zhong yao si fen san zhi liao jiao qi 47 li [47 cases of foot qi (athlete's foot) treated with four powdered Chinese drugs]."

50. Cui Yunbao et al., "Jiao qi bing kao shi ji qi yi yi [The importance of original-forms analyzing of foot qi disease]," 155.

51. Ibid., 156.

52. In his memoirlike novel *Lost Names*, based on his childhood experiences in occupied Korea, Richard E. Kim describes how Japanese appropriations of food commodities affected Korean families (94–95)

53. In the vanguard: Soyoung Suh, "Korean Medicine between the Local and the Universal," "From Influence to Confluence," "Herbs of Our Own Kingdom," and "*Shanghanlun* in Korea."

54. Michael Shiyung Liu, *Prescribing Colonization*, 47.

Conclusion

1. World Health Organization, *The Global Burden of Disease*, 47.

2. Julie Livingston, *Improvising Medicine*.

3. Marta Hanson, "Conceptual Blind Spots, Media Blindfolds."

4. Zengyi Chang, "The Discovery of Qinghaosu (Artemisinin) as an Effective Anti-Malaria Drug."

5. Bob Flaws, "Arguments for the Adoption of a Standard Translational Terminology," 17. See also Nigel Wiseman, "Chinese Medical Dictionaries."

6. As Sonya E. Pritzker has shown in *Living Translation*, however, there are many layers of resistance to that uniformity in practice, and alternative translations and understandings are unlikely to disappear regardless of what the WHO decides.

7. World Health Organization, *WHO International Standard Terminologies*, 163; and Li Zhen-ji, *International Standard Chinese–English Basic Nomenclature of Chinese Medicine*, 383.

8. Zhong yi yao xue ming ci shen ding wei yuan hui, *Zhong yi yao xue ming ci*, 246.

9. N. A. R. Wiseman, "Translation of Chinese Medical Terms," 5.

10. Ibid., 2.

11. Nigel Wiseman and Feng Ye, *A Practical Dictionary of Chinese Medicine*, 61, 129, 543, 383.

12. Ibid., 342.

13. Some are already adopting the kind of skepticism I endorse here; the draft glossary for the Chinese-medicine publisher Eastland Press, for example, suggests "diphtheria disorder" and "malarial disorder" for *white throat* and *nüe*, respectively, hinting that these are not exactly the same concepts as diphtheria and malaria. See www.eastlandpress.com/upload/3_pdf_1_20090331134930_1/Draft%20Gloss%20Trad.pdf.

Bibliography

Alter, Joseph S. *Asian Medicine and Globalization*. Philadelphia: University of Pennsylvania Press, 2005.

Anderson, E. N. *Food and Environment in Early and Medieval China*. Philadelphia: University of Pennsylvania Press, 2014.

Andrews, Bridie. *The Making of Modern Chinese Medicine, 1850–1960*. Honolulu: University of Hawai'i Press, 2015.

———. "Tailoring Tradition: The Impact of Modern Medicine on Traditional Chinese Medicine, 1887–1937," in *Notions et perceptions du changement en Chine*, edited by Viviane Alleton and Alexei Volkov. Paris: Collège de France, 1994.

———. "Tuberculosis and the Assimilation of Germ Theory in China, 1895–1937." *Journal of the History of Medicine and Allied Sciences* 52 (1997): 114–157.

Andrews, Bridie J., and Mary P. Sutphen, eds. *Medicine and Colonial Identity*. London: Routledge: 2003.

Apple, Rima D. *Vitamania: Vitamins in American Culture*. New Brunswick, NJ: Rutgers University Press, 1996.

Arnold, David. "British India and the 'Beriberi Problem,' 1798–1942," *Medical History* 54.3 (July 2010): 295–314.

———, ed. *Imperial Medicine and Indigenous Societies*. Manchester, UK: Manchester University Press, 1988.

Aronowitz, Robert A. "From the Patient's Angina Pectoris to the Cardiologist's Coronary Heart Disease." In *Making Sense of Illness: Science, Society, and Disease*, edited by Robert A. Aronowitz, 84–110. Cambridge, UK: Cambridge University Press, 1998.

Ashmead, Albert S. "Some Observations on Kakké, the National Disease of Japan." *University Medical Magazine* 3 (1891): 168–175.

Barfield, Thomas J. *The Perilous Frontier: Nomadic Empires and China.* Cambridge, MA: Basil Blackwell, 1989.

Barnes, Linda. *Needles, Herbs, Gods, and Ghosts: China, Healing, and the West to 1848.* Cambridge, MA: Harvard University Press, 2005.

Bartholomew, James R. *The Formation of Science in Japan: Building a Research Tradition.* New Haven, CT: Yale University Press, 1989.

Bay, Alexander R. *Beriberi in Modern Japan: The Making of a National Disease.* Rochester, NY: University of Rochester Press, 2012.

Beasley, W. G. *The Meiji Restoration.* Stanford, CA: Stanford University Press, 1972.

Benedict, Carol. *Bubonic Plague in Nineteenth-Century China.* Stanford, CA: Stanford University Press, 1996.

Bennett, Judith A. "Germs or Rations? Beriberi and the Japanese Labor Experiment in Colonial Fiji and Queensland." *Pacific Studies* 24.3/4 (2001): 1–17.

Bensky, Dan, and Randall Barolet. *Chinese Herbal Medicine: Formulas & Strategies.* Seattle, WA: Eastland Press, 1990.

Bensky, Dan, Steven Clavey, and Erich Stöger, eds. *Chinese Herbal Medicine: Materia Medica,* 3rd ed. Seattle, WA: Eastland Press, 2004.

"Beri-Beri (Kakké) in the United States." *Sei-I-Kwai Medical Journal* (Tokyo) 6.2 (1887): 47–48.

Beukers, H., A. M. Luyendijk-Elshout, M. E. van Opstall, and F. Vos, *Red-Hair Medicine: Dutch–Japanese Medical Relations.* Amsterdam: Rodopi, 1991.

Bokenkamp, Stephen R. "Ko Hung." In *The Indiana Companion to Traditional Chinese Literature,* vol. 1., edited by William H. Nienhauser Jr., 481–482. Bloomington: Indiana University Press, 1986.

Bol, Peter K. "Government, Society and State: On the Political Visions of Ssu-ma Kuang and Wang An-shih." In *Ordering the World: Approaches to State and Society in Sung Dynasty China,* edited by Robert P. Hymes and Conrad Schirokauer, 128–192. Berkeley: University of California Press, 1993.

Bowers, John Z. *Medical Education in Japan, from Chinese Medicine to Western Medicine.* New York: Hoeber, 1965.

———. *Western Medical Pioneers in Feudal Japan.* Baltimore, MD: Johns Hopkins University Press, 1970.

————. *When the Twain Meet: The Rise of Western Medicine in Japan.* Baltimore, MD: Johns Hopkins University Press, 1980.

Bown, Stephen R. *Scurvy: How a Surgeon, a Mariner and a Gentleman Solved the Greatest Medical Mystery of the Age of Sail.* Chichester, UK: Summersdale, 2003.

Brook, Timothy. *The Confusions of Pleasure: Commerce and Culture in Ming China.* Berkeley: University of California Press, 1998.

Bruyn, George W., and Charles M. Poser. *The History of Tropical Neurology: Nutritional Disorders.* Canton, MA: Science History Publications, 2003.

Burnham, John C. "American Medicine's Golden Age: What Happened to It?" *Science* New Series 215. 4539 (March 19, 1982): 1474–1479.

Burns, Susan L. "Contemplating Places: The Hospital as Modern Experience in Meiji Japan." In *New Directions in the Study of Meiji Japan,* edited by Helen Hardacre and Adam L. Kern, 702–718. Leiden: Brill, 1994.

Campany, Robert Ford. *To Live as Long as Heaven and Earth: A Translation and Study of Ge Hong's Traditions of Divine Transcendents.* Berkeley and Los Angeles: University of California Press, 2002.

Carpenter, Kenneth J. *Beriberi, White Rice, and Vitamin B: A Disease, a Cause, and a Cure.* Berkeley: University of California Press, 2000.

————. *The History of Scurvy and Vitamin C.* Cambridge, UK: Cambridge University Press, 1986.

Carter, K. Codell. "The Germ Theory, Beriberi, and the Deficiency Theory of Disease." *Medical History* 21 (1977): 119–136.

————. *The Rise of Causal Concepts of Disease: Case Histories.* Burlington, VT: Ashgate, 2003.

Chang, Chia-feng. "Aspects of Smallpox and Its Significance in Chinese History." PhD dissertation, SOAS, University of London, 1996.

Chang, Terence, Guo Zheng, Tony Chiu Wai Leung, Takeshi Kanehiro, Fengyi Zhang, Yong You, and Zhen Zhang. *Red Cliff.* DVD. Directed by John Woo. Los Angeles: Magnolia Home Entertainment, 2010.

Chang, Zengyi. "The Discovery of Qinghaosu (Artemisinin) as an Effective Anti-Malaria Drug: a Unique China Story." *Science China: Life Sciences* 59.1 (January 2016): 81–88.

Chao Yuanfang. "Zhu bing yuan hou lun [Sources and symptoms of all disease]." 610. In *Zhu bing yuan hou lun jiao zhu,* edited by Ding Guangdi. Beijing: Renmin weisheng chubanshe, 2000.

Chao Yüan-ling. *Medicine and Society in Late Imperial China: A Study of Physicians in Suzhou, 1600–1850*. New York: Peter Lang, 2009.

Che Ruoshui. *Jiao qi ji* [Foot qi collectanea]. 1274. Taipei: Taiwan shangwu yinshuguan, 1983.

Chen Bangxian. *Zhong guo yi xue shi* [The history of Chinese medicine]. Shanghai: Shanghai yixue shuju, 1929.

Chen Cheng, Pei Zongyuan, and Chen Shiwen. *Tai ping hui min he ji ju fang* [Formulary of the imperial pharmacy of the Great Peace and Prosperous State era]. 1110. Edited by Chen Qingping and Chen Bing'ou. Beijing: Zhongguo Zhongyiyao chubanshe: 1996.

Chen Shengkun. *Zhong guo chuan tong yi xue shi* [History of Chinese Traditional Medicine]. Taibei: Shi bao, 1979.

Chia, Lucille. *Printing for Profit: The Commercial Publishers of Jianyang, Fujian (11th–17th centuries)*. Cambridge, MA: Harvard University Press, 2002.

Chien, Cecilia Lee-fang. *Salt and State: An Annotated Translation of the Songshi Salt Monopoly Treatise*. Ann Arbor: Center for Chinese Studies at the University of Michigan, 2004.

Clunas, Craig. *Superfluous Things: Material Culture and Social Status in Early Modern China*. Urbana: University of Illinois Press, 1991.

Confucius. *The Analects (Lun yü)*. Translated by D. C. Lau. New York: Penguin Books, 1979.

Cook, N. D. *Born to Die: Disease and New World Conquest*. Cambridge, UK: Cambridge University Press, 1998.

Cooter, Roger. "The Life of a Disease?" *The Lancet* 375.9709 (January 9, 2010): 111–112.

———. "Neural Veils and the Will to Historical Critique: Why Historians of Science Need to Take the Neuro-Turn Seriously," *Isis* 105.1 (2014): 145–154.

Cousland, P.B. "Medical Nomenclature in China." *China Medical Missionary Journal* 19.2 (1905): 53–55.

Cousland, Philip B. "Notes on the Occurrence of Beri-Beri or Kakké at Swatow." *China Medical Missionary Journal* 2.2 (1888): 51–55.

Crosby, Alfred W. *Ecological Imperialism: The Biological Expansion of Europe 900–1900*. Cambridge, UK: Cambridge University Press, 1986.

Cui Yunbao et al. "Jiao qi bing kao shi ji qi yi yi [Importance of original-forms analyzing of foot qi disease]." *Liaoning Zhongyiyao daxue xuebao* 17.1 (January 2015): 155–157.

Cullen, Christopher. "*Yi'an* (Case Statements): The Origins of a Genre of Chinese Medical Literature," in *Innovation in Chinese Medicine*, edited by Elisabeth Hsu, 297–323. Cambridge, UK: Cambridge University Press, 2001.

Cunningham, Andrew. "Identifying Disease in the Past: Cutting the Gordian Knot." *Asclepio* 54.1 (2002): 13–34.

———. "Transforming Plague: The Laboratory and the Identity of Infectious Disease," chapter 7 in *The Laboratory Revolution in Medicine*, edited by Andrew Cunningham and Perry Williams. Cambridge, UK: Cambridge University Press, 1992.

Cuppage, Francis E. *James Cook and the Conquest of Scurvy*. Westport, CT: Greenwood Press, 1994.

Curtin, Philip. *Disease and Empire: The Health of European Troops in the Conquest of Africa*. Cambridge, UK: Cambridge University Press, 1998.

Dai Yuanli. *Mi chuan zheng zhi yao jue ji lei fang* [Secretly, orally transmitted methods for diagnosis and treatment, plus formulas arranged by category]. 1441. Beijing: Zhongguo Zhongyiyao chubanshe, 1998.

———. *Tui qiu shi yi* [In search of the master's meaning]. Before 1405. Edited by Zuo Yanfu. Nanjing: Jiangsu kexue jishu chubanshe, 1984.

DeBevoise, Ken. *Agents of Apocalypse: Epidemic Diseases in the Colonial Philippines*. Princeton, NJ: Princeton University Press, 1995.

Despeux, Catherine. "The System of the Five Circulatory Phases and the Six Seasonal Influences (*wuyun liuqi*), a Source of Innovation in Medicine under the Song (960–1279)." In *Innovation in Chinese Medicine*, edited by Elisabeth Hsu, 121–165. Cambridge, UK: Cambridge University Press, 2001.

Diamond, Jared. *Guns, Germs and Steel: The Fates of Human Societies*. New York: Norton, 1999.

Ding Xiaolin and Tan Hongjun, "Jiao qi yao wu de yan jiu gai kuang," *Chongqing Zhongcaoyao yanjiu* 2.1 (December 2010): 52–57.

Dong Ji. *Jiao qi zhi fa zong yao* [Comprehensive essentials for treating foot qi]. 1085. In *Si ku quan shu*. 738: 417–437. Shanghai: Shanghai guji chubanshe, 1987.

Dong Su. *Qi xiao liang fang* [Excellent formulas of miraculous efficacy]. 1471. Modern edition edited by K. E. Jia. Beijing: Zhongguo Zhongyiyao chubanshe, 1995.

Ebrey, Patricia. "The Response of the Sung State to Popular Funeral Practices." In *Religion and Society in T'ang and Sung China*, edited by

Patricia Ebrey and Peter N. Gregory, 209–239. Honolulu: University of Hawai'i Press, 1993.

Ebrey, Patricia Buckley, and Maggie Bickford, eds. *Emperor Huizong and Late Northern Song China: The Politics of Culture and the Culture of Politics.* Cambridge, MA, and London: Harvard University Asia Center, 2006.

Elman, Benjamin. *A Cultural History of Civil Examinations in Late Imperial China.* Berkeley: University of California Press, 2000.

———. *On Their Own Terms: Science in China, 1550–1900.* Cambridge, MA: Harvard University Press, 2005.

Elvin, Mark. *The Retreat of the Elephants: An Environmental History of China.* New Haven, CT: Yale University Press, 2004.

Evans, Hughes. "Losing Touch: The Controversy over the Introduction of Blood Pressure Instruments into Medicine." *Technology and Culture* 34.4 (1993): 784–807.

Faber, Knud. *Nosography: The Evolution of Clinical Medicine in Modern Times.* New York: Paul B. Hoeber, 1930.

Fan Ka-Wai. "*Jiao Qi* Disease in Medieval China." *The American Journal of Chinese Medicine* 32.6 (2004): 999–1011.

———. "The Period of Division and the Tang Period." Chapter 3 In *Chinese Medicine and Healing: An Illustrated History*, edited by TJ Hinrichs and Linda L. Barnes, 65–96. Cambridge, MA: Belknap Press, 2013.

Fan Xingzhun. *Zhong guo bing shi xin yi* [New readings in the history of disease in China]. Beijing: Zhongyi guji chubanshe, 1989.

———. *Zhong guo yi xue shi lue* [Summary of the history of Chinese medicine]. Beijing: Zhongyi guji chubanshe, 1986.

"The Far Eastern Association of Tropical Medicine," *The Lancet* 175.4522 (April 30, 1910): 1227–1230.

Flaws, Bob. "Arguments for the Adoption of a Standard Translational Terminology in the Study & Practice of Chinese Medicine in the English-Speaking World." *American Acupuncturist* 37 (Fall 2006): 16–27.

Francks, Penelope. "Inconspicuous Consumption: Sake, Beer, and the Birth of the Consumer in Japan." *Journal of Asian Studies* 68.1 (February 2009): 135–164.

———. "Simple Pleasures: Food Consumption in Japan and the Global Comparison of Living Standards." *Journal of Global History* 8.1 (March 2013): 95–116.

Franke, Herbert, and Denis Twitchett, eds. *Alien Regimes and Border States, 907–1368.* Vol. 6 of *The Cambridge History of China.* Cambridge, UK: Cambridge University Press, 1994.

Fu Lisheng. *Jiao qi zheng jing yan liang fang* [Excellent tried-and-true formulas for foot *qi* syndrome]. 1906. First edition held in the library of the Zhongyi kexue yuan in Beijing.

Fu Youfeng, "Jiao qi ben yi yu xian shu yi shi hua [Historical discussion of plague and the original meaning of foot qi]. *Nanjing Zhongyiyao daxue xuebao* 7,1 (March 2006): 25–31.

Furth, Charlotte. "Becoming Alternative? Modern Transformations of Chinese Medicine in China and the United States." *Canadian Bulletin of Medical History* 28.1 (2011): 5–41.

———. *A Flourishing Yin: Gender in China's Medical History, 960–1665.* Berkeley, Los Angeles, and London: University of California Press, 1999.

Furth, Charlotte, and Angela Ki Che Leung, eds. *Health and Hygiene in Chinese East Asia: Politics and Publics in the Long Twentieth Century.* Durham, NC: Duke University Press, 2010.

Ge Hong. *Zhou hou bei ji fang* [Emergency formulas to keep up one's sleeve]. Late third century/early fourth century. In *Bao pu zi nei pian, Zhou hou bei ji fang jin yi,* edited by Mei Quanxi et al. Beijing: Zhongguo Zhongyiyao chubanshe, 1997.

Goble, Andrew Edmund. *Confluences of Medicine in Medieval Japan: Buddhist Healing, Chinese Knowledge, Islamic Formulas, and Wounds of War.* Honolulu: University of Hawai'i Press, 2011.

Goldschmidt, Asaf. "Commercializing Medicine or Benefiting the People: The First Public Pharmacy in China." *Science in Context* 21.3 (September 2008): 311–350.

———. *The Evolution of Chinese Medicine: Song Dynasty 960–1200.* London: Routledge, 2011.

———. "Huizong's Impact on Medicine and Public Health." In *Emperor Huizong and Late Northern Song China: The Politics of Culture and the Culture of Politics,* edited by Patricia Buckley Ebrey and Maggie Bickford, 275–323. Cambridge, MA, and London: Harvard University Asia Center, 2006.

Gong Tingxian. *Wan bing hui chun* [Restoring health from the myriad disorders]. 1587. Beijing: Renmin weisheng chubanshe, 1984.

Grant, Joanna. *A Chinese Physician: Wang Ji and the Stone Mountain Medical Case Histories*. London: RoutledgeCurzon, 2003.

Greene, Jeremy A. *Prescribing by Numbers: Drugs and the Definition of Disease*. Baltimore, MD: Johns Hopkins University Press, 2008.

Guangdong Province Academy of Traditional Chinese Medicine, eds. *Zhong yi lin chuang xin bian* [Newly edited volume on clinical Traditional Chinese Medicine]. Guangzhou: Guangdong renmin chubanshe, 1972.

Haensch, Stephanie, Raffaella Bianucci, Michel Signoli, Minoarisoa Rajerison, Michael Schultz, Sacha Kacki, Marco Vermunt, et al. "Distinct Clones of *Yersinia Pestis* Caused the Black Death." *PLoS Pathogens* 6.10 (2010).

Hansen, Valerie. *The Open Empire: A History of China to 1600*. New York: W. W. Norton, 2000.

Hanson, Marta. "Conceptual Blind Spots, Media Blindfolds: The Case of SARS and Traditional Chinese Medicine." In *Health and Hygiene in Chinese East Asia*, edited by Angela Ki Che Leung and Charlotte Furth, 228–254. Durham, NC: Duke University Press, 2010.

———. "Northern Purgatives, Southern Restoratives: Ming Medical Regionalism." *Asian Medicine: Tradition and Modernity* 2.2 (2006): 115–170.

———. *Speaking of Epidemics in Chinese Medicine: Disease and the Geographic Imagination in Late Imperial China*. London: RoutledgeCurzon, 2011.

Harrison, Mark. *Climates and Constitutions: Health, Race, Environment and British Imperialism in India, 1600–1850*. Oxford, UK: Oxford University Press, 2003.

———. *Disease and the Modern World: 1500 to the Present Day*. Cambridge, UK: Polity, 2004.

Heinrich, Larissa N. *The Afterlife of Images: Translating the Pathological Body between China and the West*. Durham, NC: Duke University Press, 2008.

———. "How China Became the 'Cradle of Smallpox': Transformations in Discourse, 1726–2002." *Positions: East Asia Cultures Critique* 15.1 (2007): 7–34.

Hicks, Angela. *Discovering Holistic Health: Principles of Chinese Medicine*. London: Singing Dragon, 2013.

Hinrichs, TJ. "Governance through Medical Texts and the Role of Print," in *Knowledge and Text Production in an Age of Print: China, 900–1400*, edited by Lucille Chia and Hilde De Weerdt, 217–238. Leiden: Brill, 2011.

———. "The Medical Transforming of Governance and Southern Customs in Song Dynasty China (960–1279 C.E.)." PhD dissertation, Harvard University, 2003.

———, "The Song and Jin Periods," in *Chinese Medicine and Healing: An Illustrated History*, edited by TJ Hinrichs and Linda Barnes. Cambridge, MA: The Belknap Press, 2013.

Hinrichs, TJ, and Linda Barnes, eds. *Chinese Medicine and Healing: An Illustrated History.* Cambridge, MA: The Belknap Press, 2013.

Hong Hai. *The Theory of Chinese Medicine: A Modern Explanation.* London: Imperial College Press, 2014.

"Hong Kong Acting Colonial Surgeon's Report for 1895." Hong Kong Government Reports Online (1853–1941). Retrieved on March 3, 2008, from http://sunzi1.lib.hku.hk/hkgro/index.jsp.

Hou Xiangchuan et al. *Nutritional Studies in Shanghai.* Shanghai: Henry Lester Medical Institute, 1940.

Hsu, Elisabeth. "Tactility and the Body in Early Chinese Medicine," *Science in Context* 18 (2005): 7–34.

———. *The Transmission of Chinese Medicine.* Cambridge, UK: Cambridge University Press, 1999.

Hu Dongpei. *Traditional Chinese Medicine: Theory and Principles.* Berlin and Beijing: deGruyter and Tsinghua University Press, 2016.

Hu Ling. "Lao Zhong yi tui jian de zhi liao jiao qi pian fang [Folk prescriptions for treating foot qi (athlete's foot), recommended by senior Chinese-medicine doctors]." *Nongjia zhi you* 6 (2014): 41.

Huang Di nei jing su wen: An Annotated Translation of Huang Di's Inner Classic—Basic Questions. Translated and edited by Paul U. Unschuld and Hermann Tessenow in collaboration with Zheng Jinsheng. Berkeley: University of California Press, 2011.

Huang, H. T. *Science and Civilisation in China. Vol. 6: Biology and Biological Technology, Part V: Fermentations and Food Science.* Cambridge, UK: Cambridge University Press, 2000.

Huang di nei jing su wen [Basic questions of the Yellow Emperor's inner canon]. ca. 1st century BC. Beijing: Xueyuan chubanshe, 2002.

Hymes, Robert. "Not Quite Gentlemen? Doctors in Sung and Yuan." *Chinese Science* 8 (1987): 9–76.

Imamura Ryōan. *Kakke kōyō* [Essentials of foot qi]. 1861. Tokyo: Suhachiya Shinbei, 1864.

Ishiguro Tadanori. *Kakke ron* [Foot qi treatise]. Tokyo: Shimamura Yoshimatsu, 1878.

Itokawa, Yoshinori. "Kanehiro Takaki (1849–1920): A Biographical Sketch." *Journal of Nutrition* 106. 5 (1976): 583–588.

Jannetta, Ann Bowman. *Epidemics and Mortality in Early Modern Japan.* Princeton, NJ: Princeton University Press, 1987.

Jeanselme, Edouard. *Le Béribéri.* Paris: Masson, 1906.

"Jiao qi bing zen me zhi liao? [How do you treat foot qi disease?]," Baidu Zhidao. Retrieved on June 26, 2013, from http://zhidao.baidu.com/question/215675.html.

Jiang Guan. *Ming yi lei an* [Categorized case records of famous doctors]. 1549. Taibei: Hongye shuju, 1979.

Johnston, William. *The Modern Epidemic: A History of Tuberculosis in Japan.* Cambridge, MA: Harvard University Press, 1995.

Jones, David S. "Virgin Soils Revisited." *The William and Mary Quarterly* LX.4 (2003): 703–742.

Kamminga, Harmke, and Andrew Cunningham, eds. *The Science and Culture of Nutrition, 1840–1940.* Atlanta, GA: Rodopi, 1995.

Kaptchuk, Ted J. *The Web That Has No Weaver: Understanding Chinese Medicine.* Chicago: McGraw-Hill, 2000.

Karchmer, Eric I. "Chinese Medicine in Action: On the Postcoloniality of Medical Practice in China." *Medical Anthropology* 29.3 (2010): 226–252.

———. "Slow Medicine: How Chinese Medicine Became Efficacious Only for Chronic Conditions." In *Historical Epistemology and the Making of Modern Chinese Medicine,* edited by Howard Chiang, 188–216. Manchester, UK: Manchester University Press, 2015.

Keegan, David Joseph. "The 'Huang-ti-nei-ching': The Structure of the Compilation; the Significance of the Structure." PhD dissertation, University of California, Berkeley, 1988.

Kieschnick, John, "Buddhist Vegetarianism in China." In *Of Tripod and Palate: Food, Politics, and Religion in Traditional China,* edited by Roel Sterckx. New York: Palgrave MacMillan, 2004.

Kim, Richard E. *Lost Names: Scenes from a Korean Boyhood.* Berkeley: University of California Press, 1998.

Kipling, Rudyard. "The White Man's Burden." In *Empire Writing: An Anthology of Colonial Literature 1870–1918*, edited by Elleke Boehmer, 481–483. Oxford, UK: Oxford University Press, 1998.

Knechtges, David. "Gradually Entering the Realm of Delight: Food and Drink in Early Medieval China." *Journal of the American Oriental Society* 117.2 (1997): 229–239.

Kohn, Livia. *Chinese Healing Exercises: The Tradition of Daoyin*. Honolulu: University of Hawai'i Press, 2008.

Kohn, Livia, and Yoshinobu Sakade, eds. *Taoist Meditation and Longevity Techniques*. Ann Arbor, MI: Center for Chinese Studies, 1989.

Kuriyama, Shigehisa. "Epidemics, Weather, and Contagion in Traditional Chinese Medicine." In *Contagion: Perspectives from Pre-Modern Societies*, edited by Lawrence I. Conrad and Dominik Wujastyk, 3–22. Burlington, VT: Ashgate, 2000.

———. *The Expressiveness of the Body and the Divergence of Greek and Chinese Medicine*. Cambridge, MA: MIT Press, 1999.

Lackner, Michael, Iwo Amelung, and Joachim Kurtz, eds. *New Terms for New Ideas: Western Knowledge and Lexical Change in Late Imperial China*. Sinica Leidensia, 52. Leiden, Boston, and Köln: Brill, 2001.

Latour, Bruno. *The Pasteurization of France*. Cambridge, MA: Harvard University Press, 1988.

Lee, Seung-joon. *Gourmets in the Land of Famine: The Culture and Politics of Rice in Modern Canton*. Stanford, CA: Stanford University Press, 2011.

———. "The Patriot's Scientific Diet: Nutritional Science and Dietary Reform Campaigns in China, 1910s–1950s." *Modern Asian Studies* 49.6 (November 2015): 1808–1839.

Lee, Thomas H. C. "Sung Schools and Education before Chu Hsi." In *Neo-Confucian Education: The Formative Stage*, edited by William Theodore deBary and John W. Chaffee, 105–136. Berkeley: University of California Press, 1989.

LeFanu, James. *The Rise and Fall of Modern Medicine*. New York: Carroll & Graf Publishers, 1999.

Lei, Sean Hsiang-lin. *Neither Donkey nor Horse: Medicine in the Struggle over China's Modernity*. Chicago: University of Chicago Press, 2014.

Leung, Angela Ki Che. "Japanese Medical Texts in Chinese on Kakké in the Tokugawa and Early Meiji Periods." In *Antiquarianism, Language, and Medical Philology: From Early Modern to Modern Sino-Japanese*

Medical Discourses, edited by Benjamin A. Elman, 163–185. Leiden: Brill, 2015.

———. *Leprosy in China*. New York: Columbia University Press, 2009.

———. "Medical Instruction and Popularization in Ming-Qing China." *Late Imperial China* 24.1 (2003): 130–152.

———. "Organized Medicine in Ming-Qing China: State and Private Medical Institutions in the Lower Yangzi Region," *Late Imperial China* 8.1 (1987): 134–166.

———. "Zhong guo ma feng bing gai nian yan bian de li shi [The history of the evolution of concepts of *ma feng* disease in China]." *Zhongyang yanjiuyuan lishi yuyan yanjiusuo jikan* 70.2 (1999): 399–438.

Levenstein, Harvey. *Revolution at the Table: The Transformation of the American Diet*. Oxford, UK: Oxford University Press, 1988.

Li Chan. *Yi xue ru men* [Introduction to the study of medicine]. 1575. Edited by Jin Yanli et al. Beijing: Zhongguo Zhongyiyao chubanshe, 1995.

Li Dong-yuan. *Treatise on the Spleen and Stomach*. Translated by Yang Shou-zhong and Li Jian-yong. Boulder, CO: Blue Poppy Press, 1997.

Li Gao. *Yi xue fa ming*. [Clarifying the study of medicine]. 1251. In *Xu xiu si ku quan shu*, v. 1005: 530–562. Shanghai: Shanghai guji chubanshe, 1995.

Li Jingwei and Deng Tietao, et al., eds. *Zhong yi da ci dian* [Dictionary of Chinese Medicine]. Beijing: Renmin weisheng chubanshe, 1995.

Li Jingwei and Lin Zhaogeng. *Zhong guo yi xue tong shi: gu dai juan* [A general history of Chinese medicine: volume on ancient times]. vol. 1. Edited by Chen Minzhang. Beijing: Renmin weisheng chubanshe, 1999.

Li Shizhen. *Ben cao gang mu* [Systematic materia medica]. Composed 1587, printed 1596. 4 volumes. Beijing: Renmin weisheng chubanshe, 1975.

Li Yongcui. *Zheng zhi hui bu* [Collected supplements to the (Standards for) diagnosis and therapy]. 1687. Edited by Wu Wei. Beijing: Zhongguo Zhongyiyao chubanshe, 1999.

Li Zhen-ji, ed. *International Standard Chinese–English Basic Nomenclature of Chinese Medicine*. Beijing: People's Medical Publishing House, 2014.

Liao Yuqun. "Guan yu Zhong guo gu dai de jiao qi bing ji qi li shi de yan jiu [Research on the history of foot qi disease in ancient China]." *Studies in the History of Natural Sciences* 19, 3 (2000): 206–221.

————. "Ji zai yu quan shi—Ri ben jiao qi bing shi de zai jian tao [Records and explanatory notes—reinvestigating the history of foot *qi* disease in Japan]." *New History* 12.4 (2001): 121–154.

————. "Mai fan nan jue—Takaki Kanehiro [Takaki Kanehiro, barley baron]." *Gu jin lun heng*, 6 (2001): 90–103.

Liao Yuqun, Fu Fang, and Zheng Jinsheng. *Zhong guo ke xue ji shu shi, yi xue juan* [History of Chinese science and technology, medicine volume]. Beijing: Kexue chubanshe, 1998.

Liu Chenweng. *Xu xi ji* [Collectanea of Xu xi (Liu Chenweng)]. Late thirteenth century. In *Si ku quan shu*, vol. 1186. Shanghai: Shanghai guji chubanshe, 1987.

Liu, Michael Shiyung. *Prescribing Colonization: The Role of Medical Practices and Policies in Japan-Ruled Taiwan, 1895–1945*. Ann Arbor, MI: Association for Asian Studies, 2009.

Livingston, Julie. *Improvising Medicine: An African Oncology Ward in an Emerging Cancer Epidemic*. Durham, NC: Duke University Press, 2012.

Lloyd, Geoffrey, and Nathan Sivin. *The Way and the Word: Science and Medicine in Early China and Greece*. New Haven, CT: Yale University Press, 2002.

Lo, Vivienne. "The Han Period." In *Chinese Medicine and Healing: An Illustrated History*, edited by TJ Hinrichs and Linda L. Barnes, 31–64. Cambridge, MA: The Belknap Press, 2013.

————. "The Influence of *Yangsheng* Culture on Early Chinese Medical Theory." PhD dissertation, University of London, 1998.

————, ed. *Medieval Chinese Medicine: The Dunhuang Medical Manuscripts*. London: RoutledgeCurzon, 2005.

Lock, Margaret. *East Asian Medicine in Urban Japan: Varieties of Medical Experience*. Berkeley: University of California Press, 1980.

Lou Ying. *Yi xue gang mu* [The systematic study of medicine]. 1565. Edited by Gao Dengying and Lu Zhaolin. 2 vols. Beijing: Renmin weisheng chubanshe, 1987.

Low, Morris. *Building a Modern Japan: Science, Technology, and Medicine in the Meiji Era and Beyond*. New York: Palgrave Macmillan, 2005.

Lu Gwei-djen and Joseph Needham. "A Contribution to the History of Chinese Dietetics," *Isis* 42.1 (April 1951), 13–20.

Luesink, David. "State Power, Governmentality, and the (Mis)Remembrance of Chinese Medicine." In *Historical Epistemology and the Making of Modern Chinese Medicine*, edited by Howard Chiang, 160–187. Manchester, UK: Manchester University Press, 2015.

Luo Zhufeng, chief ed. *Han yu da ci dian* [The Great Dictionary of the Chinese Language]. 10 vols. Shanghai: Hanyu da cidian chubanshe, 2001.

Ma Jixing. *Zhong yi wen xian xue* [The study of Chinese medical documents]. Shanghai: Shanghai kexue jishu chubanshe, 1990.

MacLeod, Roy, and Milton Lewis, eds. *Disease, Medicine, and Empire: Perspectives on Western Medicine and the Experience of European Expansion*. London and New York: Routledge, 1988.

MacPherson, Kerrie L. "Cholera in China, 1820–1930: An Aspect of the Internationalization of Infectious Disease." In *Sediments of Time: Environment and Society in Chinese History*, edited by Mark Elvin and Liu Ts'ui-jung, 487–519. Cambridge, UK: Cambridge University Press, 1998.

Malcolmson, John Grant. *A Practical Essay on the History and Treatment of Beriberi*. Madras: Vespery Mission Press, 1835.

Manson, Patrick. *Tropical Diseases: A Manual of the Diseases of Warm Climates*. New York: William Wood, 1898.

Marks, Harry. *The Progress of Experiment: Science and Therapeutic Reform in the U.S., 1900–1990*. Cambridge, UK: Cambridge University Press, 1997.

Marmé, Michael. *Suzhou: Where the Goods of All the Provinces Converge*. Stanford, CA: Stanford University Press, 2005.

McCollum, Elmer Verner. *A History of Nutrition: The Sequence of Ideas in Nutrition Investigations*. Boston: Houghton Mifflin, 1957.

McDermott, Joseph P. *A Social History of the Chinese Book: Books and Literati Culture in Late Imperial China*. Hong Kong: Hong Kong University Press, 2006.

McKeown, Thomas. *The Role of Medicine: Dream, Mirage, or Nemesis?* London: The Nuffield Provincial Hospitals Trust, 1976.

McMillen, Christian. *Discovering Tuberculosis: A Global History, 1900 to the Present*. New Haven, CT: Yale University Press, 2015.

McNeill, J. R. *Mosquito Empires: Ecology and War in the Greater Caribbean*. Cambridge, UK: Cambridge University Press, 2010.

McNeill, William H. *Plagues and Peoples*. New York: Anchor Books, 1976.

Mencius, *The Works of Mencius*. Translated by James Legge. New York: Dover, 1970.

Meng Shen. *Shi liao ben cao* [Materia medica for food therapy]. 713–741. Modern edition edited by Xie Haizhou et al. Beijing: Renmin weisheng chubanshe, 1984.

Mukherjee, Siddhartha. *The Emperor of All Maladies: A Biography of Cancer.* New York: Scribner, 2011.

Nakamura, Ellen Gardner. *Practical Pursuits: Takano Choei, Takahashi Keisaku, and Western Medicine in Nineteenth-Century Japan.* Cambridge, MA: Harvard University Asia Center, 2005.

Oberländer, Christian. "The Rise of Scientific Medicine in Japan: Beriberi as the Driving Force in the Quest for Specific Causes and the Introduction of Bacteriology." *Historia Scientiarum* 13.3 (March 2004): 176–199.

Ohnuki-Tierney, Emiko. *Rice as Self: Japanese Identities through Time.* Princeton, NJ: Princeton University Press, 1993.

Ohomori, Kenta. "Studies on the Cause and Treatment of Beri-Beri in Japan." *Japan Medical World* 3.11 (1923): 231–238.

Okamoto Shōan. *Kakke bunrui hen* [The book of categories of *kakke*]. Tokyo, 1812.

Okanishi Tamehito, *Song yi qian yi ji kao* [Studies of medical books of the Song dynasty and earlier]. Beijing: Renmin weisheng chubanshe, 1958.

Oseki, Sakae. "Beriberi Like Disease in Mammalian Animals," *The Japan Medical World* 1 (May–December 1921), 6–11.

Otsuka, Yasuo. "Chinese Traditional Medicine in Japan," in *Asian Medical Systems*, edited by Charles Leslie.. Berkeley: University of California Press, 1976.

Packard, Randall. *The Making of a Tropical Disease: A Short History of Malaria.* Baltimore, MD: Johns Hopkins University Press, 2007.

Peitzman, Steven J. "From Bright's Disease to End-Stage Renal Disease." In *Framing Disease: Studies in Cultural History*, edited by Charles E. Rosenberg and Janet Golden. New Brunswick, NJ: Rutgers University Press, 1997.

Padilla, Roberto. "Science, Nurses, Physicians and Disease: The Role of Medicine in the Construction of a Modern Japanese Identity." PhD dissertation, Ohio State University, 2009.

Peng, Mu. "The Doctor's Body: Embodiment and Multiplicity of Chinese Medical Knowledge." *East Asian Science, Technology and Medicine* 25 (2006): 27–46, 1812.

Peng Wei. "Jiao qi bing, xing bing, tian hua: Han dai yi wen ji bing de kao cha [Beriberi, venereal disease, smallpox: an investigation of whether or not these diseases existed in the Han Dynasty]." *Zhejiang xuekan* 2 (2015): 54–70.

Porkert, Manfred. *The Theoretical Foundations of Chinese Medicine: Systems of Correspondence.* Cambridge, MA: MIT Press, 1974.

Porter, Roy. *The Greatest Benefit to Mankind: A Medical History of Humanity.* New York: Norton, 1997.

Powell, J. M. *Bring out Your Dead: The Great Plague of Yellow Fever in Philadelphia in 1793.* Philadelphia: University of Pennsylvania Press, 1993.

Pregadio, Fabrizio. "Chao Yuanfang." In *Encyclopaedia of the History of Science, Technology, and Medicine in Non-Western Cultures*, edited by Helaine Selin, 87–88. Berlin: Kluwer Academic, 1997.

———. *Great Clarity: Daoism and Alchemy in Early Medieval China.* Stanford, CA: Stanford University Press, 2002.

Pritzker, Sonya E. *Living Translation: Language and the Search for Resonance in U.S. Chinese Medicine.* New York: Berghahn Books, 2014.

Qiu Peiran, ed. *Zhong guo yi ji da ci dian* [The great dictionary of Chinese medical texts]. 2 vols. Shanghai: Shanghai kexue jishu chubanshe, 2002.

Rawski, Evelyn S. "Economic and Social Foundations of Late Imperial Culture." In *Popular Culture in Late Imperial China*, edited by David Johnson, Andrew J. Nathan, and Evelyn S. Rawski, 3–33. Berkeley: University of California Press, 1985.

Read, Bernard E. *Famine Foods Listed in the Chiu Huang Pen Ts'ao Giving Their Identity, Nutritional Values and Notes on Their Preparation.* Shanghai: Henry Lester Institute of Medical Research, 1946.

Rodwell, Victor W. *Harper's Illustrated Biochemistry.* New York: Lange Medical Books/McGraw-Hill, 2003.

Rogaski, Ruth. *Hygienic Modernity: Meanings of Health and Disease in Treaty-Port China.* Berkeley and Los Angeles: University of California Press, 2004.

Rogers, Naomi. *Polio Wars: Sister Kenny and the Golden Age of American Medicine.* Oxford, UK: Oxford University Press, 2013.

Rose, Nikolas. "The Human Sciences in a Biological Age." *Theory, Culture & Society* 30.1 (2013): 3–34.

Rosenberg, Charles E. "Framing Disease: Illness, Society, and History." In *Framing Disease: Studies in Cultural History*, edited by Charles Rosenberg and Janet Golden. New Brunswick, NJ: Rutgers University Press, 1997.

———. "The Tyranny of Diagnosis: Specific Entities and Individual Experience." *The Milbank Quarterly* 80,2 (2002): 237–260.

Rossabi, Morris. *China among Equals: The Middle Kingdom and Its Neighbors, 10th–14th Centuries.* Berkeley: University of California Press, 1983.

Sailey, Jay. *The Master Who Embraces Simplicity: A Study of the Philosopher Ko Hung, A.D. 283–343.* San Francisco: Chinese Materials Center, 1978.

Salguero, C. Pierce. *Translating Buddhist Medicine in Medieval China.* Philadelphia: University of Pennsylvania Press, 2014.

Sand, Jordan. "How Tokyo Invented Sushi," in *Food and the City*, edited by Dorothée Imbert. Washington, DC: Dumbarton Oaks, 2014.

Saneyoshi, Y. "On Kak'ke (Beri-Beri)." *Sei-I-Kwai Medical Journal* 20.4 (1901): 55–60.1.

Schafer, Edward H. *The Vermilion Bird: T'ang Images of the South.* Berkeley and Los Angeles: University of California Press, 1967.

Scheid, Volker. *Chinese Medicine in Contemporary China: Plurality and Synthesis.* Durham, NC: Duke University Press, 2002.

———. *Currents of Tradition in Chinese Medicine, 1626–2006.* Seattle: Eastland Press, 2007.

Scheube, B. "Die Japanische Kak-ke (Beri-beri)." *Deutsches Archiv für Klinische Medicin* (May 30, 1882): 141–202.

———. *Die Krankheiten der Warmen Länder: Ein Handbuch für ärtze.* Jena, Germany: Verlag von Gustav Fischer, 1900.

Scrinis, Gyorgy. *Nutritionism: The Science and Politics of Dietary Advice.* New York: Columbia University Press, 2010.

Semba, Richard D. *The Vitamin A Story: Lifting the Shadow of Death.* Basel: Karger, 2012.

Shanghai Academy of Traditional Chinese Medicine, eds. *Bian zheng shi zhi* [Differentiating syndromes and administering treatment]. Shanghai: Shanghai renmin chubanshe, 1972.

Shen Fu et al. *Zheng he sheng ji zong lu* [Medical encyclopedia: A sagely benefaction of the Regnant Harmony era]. Compiled 1111–1117. Taibei: Huagang chuban youxian gongsi, 1978.

Shimazono, Norio, and Eisuke Katsura. *Review of Japanese Literature on Beriberi and Thiamine.* Tokyo: Igaku Shoin, 1965.

Simmons, Duane B. "Beriberi, or the 'Kakké' of Japan." *Customs Gazette* 19 (1880): 38–76.

Sivin, Nathan. *Chinese Alchemy: Preliminary Studies.* Cambridge, MA: Harvard University Press, 1968.

————. *Health Care in Eleventh-Century China*. Cham, Switzerland: Springer, 2015.

————. "Text and Experience in Classical Chinese Medicine." In *Knowledge and the Scholarly Medical Tradition*, edited by Don Bates, 177–204. Cambridge, UK: Cambridge University Press, 1995.

————. *Traditional Medicine in Contemporary China*. Ann Arbor: Center for Chinese Studies, The University of Michigan, 1987.

Skaff, Jonathan Karam. *Sui-Tang China and Its Turko-Mongol Neighbors: Culture, Power, and Connections, 580–800*. Oxford, UK: Oxford University Press, 2012.

Smith, Paul J. "State Power and Economic Activism during the New Policies, 1068–1085: The Tea and Horse Trade and the 'Green Sprouts' Loan Policy." In *Ordering the World: Approaches to State and Society in Sung Dynasty China*, edited by Robert P. Hymes and Conrad Schirokauer, 76–127. Berkeley: University of California Press, 1993.

Somers, Robert. "The Sui Legacy." In *The Sui Dynasty*, edited by Arthur F. Wright. New York: Knopf, 1978.

Stepan, Nancy. *Eradication: Ridding the World of Diseases Forever?* Ithaca, NY: Cornell University Press, 2011.

Sterckx, Roel, ed. *Of Tripod and Palate: Food, Politics, and Religion in Traditional China*. New York: Palgrave MacMillan, 2004.

Strickmann, Michel. *Chinese Magical Medicine*, edited by Carl Bielefeldt and Bernard Faure. Stanford, CA: Stanford University Press, 2002.

Sugimoto, Masayoshi, and David L. Swain, *Science and Culture in Traditional Japan A.D. 600–1854*. Cambridge, MA: MIT Press, 1978.

Suh, Soyoung. "From Influence to Confluence: Positioning the History of Pre-Modern Korean Medicine in East Asia." *Korean Journal of Medical History* 19 (2010): 225–254.

————. "Herbs of Our Own Kingdom: Layers of the 'Local' in the Materia Medica of Early Chosŏn Korea." *Asian Medicine: Tradition and Modernity* 4.2 (2008): 395–422.

————. "Korean Medicine between the Local and the Universal: 1600–1945." PhD dissertation, UCLA, 2006.

————. "*Shanghanlun* in Korea, 1610–1945." *Asian Medicine: Tradition and Modernity* 8.1/2 (2015): 423–457.

Summers, William C. *The Great Manchurian Plague of 1910–1911: The Geopolitics of an Epidemic Disease*. New Haven, CT: Yale University Press, 2012.

Sun Simiao. "Bei ji qian jin yao fang" [Essential emergency formulas worth a thousand in gold]. ca. 650–659. In *Bei ji qian jin yao fang jiao shi*, edited by Li Jingrong. Beijing: Renmin weisheng chubanshe, 1996.

Sussman, George D. "Scientists Doing History: Central Africa and the Origins of the First Plague Pandemic," *Journal of World History* 26.2 (June 2015): 325–354.

Suzuki, Takao. *Palaeopathological and Palaeoepidemiological Study of Osseous Syphilis in Skulls of the Edo Period.* Tokyo: University of Tokyo Press, 1984.

Takaki, Kanehiro. "Japanese Navy and Army Sanitation." *Surgery, Gynecology and Obstetrics* 2 (1906): 421–440.

———. "On the Cause and Prevention of Kak'ke." *Seiikai geppo* 4, Supplement 4 (1885): 29–37.

Tamba no Yasuyori. *Ishimpō* [Formulas at the heart of medicine]. 976–984. Edited by Gao Wenzhu Beijing: Huaxia chubanshe, 1996.

Taylor, Kim. *Chinese Medicine in Early Communist China (1945–1963): Medicine of Revolution.* London and New York: RoutledgeCurzon, 2005.

Thompson, C. Michele. *Vietnamese Traditional Medicine: A Social History.* Singapore: National University of Singapore Press, 2015.

Tillman, Hoyt Cleveland, and Stephen H. West, eds. *China under Jurchen Rule: Essays on Chin Intellectual and Cultural History.* Albany: State University of New York Press, 1995.

Tsien, Tsuen-Hsuin. *Science and Civilisation in China: Vol. V. Chemistry and Chemical Technology. Part 1. Paper and Printing.* Cambridge, UK: Cambridge University Press, 1985.

Tu Ya, Yang Huimin, and Zhao Lirong. "Ying er nao xing jiao qi bing 6 li wu zhen bao dao [A report on 6 cases of misdiagnosed neurological beriberi in infants]." *Erke yaoxue zazhi* 20.1 (2014): 61–63.

Unschuld, Paul U. *Medicine in China: A History of Ideas.* Berkeley and Los Angeles: University of California Press, 1985.

Vedder, Edward B. *Beriberi.* New York: William Wood and Company, 1913.

Wan Guodong, "Ge Hong yu *Zhou hou bei ji fang.*" [Ge Hong and the *Emergency formulas to keep up one's sleeve*]. *Jiating Zhongyiyao* 5 (1998): 4.

Wang Gang. *Yue liang bei mian* [Behind the moon]. Beijing: Renmin wenxue chubanshe, 1996.

Wang Huaiyin. *Tai ping sheng hui fang* [Imperial grace formulary of the Great Peace and Prosperous State era]. 992. Beijing: Renmin weisheng chubanshe, 1982.

Wang Kentang. *Zheng zhi zhun sheng* [Standards for diagnosis and treatment]. 1602. Shanghai: Shanghai guji chubanshe, 1991.

Wang Shuo. *Yi jian fang* [Easy, concise formulas]. ca. 1191. Edited by Chao Yinci. Beijing: Renmin weisheng chubanshe, 1995.

Wang Tao. *Wai tai mi yao fang* [Arcane essentials from the imperial library]. 752. Edited by Gao Wenzhu et al. Beijing: Huaxia chubanshe, 1993.

Ware, James R. *Alchemy, Medicine, Religion in the China of A.D. 320: The Nei-p'ien of Ko Hung (Pao p'u-tzu)*. Cambridge, MA: MIT Press, 1966.

Warner, John Harley. *Against the Spirit of System: The French Impulse in Nineteenth-Century American Medicine*. Princeton, NJ: Princeton University Press, 1998.

———. *The Therapeutic Perspective: Medical Practice, Knowledge, and Identity in America, 1820–1885*. Cambridge, MA: Harvard University Press, 1986.

Watts, Sheldon. *Epidemics and History: Disease, Power, and Imperialism*. New Haven, CT: Yale University Press, 1998.

Webb, James L. A. Jr, "Malaria and the Peopling of Early Tropical Africa." *Journal of World History* 16.3 (September, 2005): 269–291.

Wei Zixiao and Nie Lifang, *Zhong yi Zhong yao shi* [The history of Chinese medicine and pharmacology]. Taibei: Wen jin chubanshe, 1994.

Wells, Matthew V. *To Die and Not Decay: Autobiography and the Pursuit of Immortality in Early China*. Ann Arbor, MI: Association for Asian Studies, 2009.

Whorton, James C. *Nature Cures: The History of Alternative Medicine in America*. Oxford, UK: Oxford University Press, 2002.

Williams, Robert R. *Toward the Conquest of Beriberi*. Cambridge, MA: Harvard University Press, 1961.

Wilms, Sabine. "The Female Body in Medieval China: A Translation and Interpretation of the 'Women's Recipes' in Sun Simiao's *Beiji qianjin yaofang*." PhD dissertation, University of Arizona, 2002.

Wilson, Adrian. "On the History of Disease-Concepts: The Case of Pleurisy," *History of Medicine* 38,3 (September 2000): 271–319.

Wiseman, N. A. R. "Translation of Chinese Medical Terms: A Source-Oriented Approach." PhD dissertation, University of Exeter, UK, 2000.

Wiseman, Nigel. "Chinese Medical Dictionaries: A Guarantee for Better Quality Literature." *Clinical Acupuncture and Oriental Medicine* 2.1 (March 2001): 36–49.

Wiseman, Nigel, and Feng Ye. *A Practical Dictionary of Chinese Medicine.* Brookline, MA: Paradigm Publications, 1998.

Wong, K. Chimin, and Wu Lien-teh. 1936. *History of Chinese Medicine,* 2nd edition. New York: AMS Press, 1973.

Worboys, Michael. "The Discovery of Colonial Malnutrition between the Wars," in *Imperial Medicine and Indigenous Societies,* edited by David Arnold, 208—25. Manchester, UK: Manchester University Press, 1988.

World Health Organization, "History of the Development of the ICD," Retrieved on March 23, 2017, from www.who.int/classifications/icd/en/HistoryOfICD.pdf.

———. *The Global Burden of Disease: 2004 Update.* Geneva: WHO Press, 2008.

———. *WHO International Standard Termonologies on Traditional Medicine in the Western Pacific Region.* Manila: WHO, 2007.

Wright, Arthur F., ed. *The Sui Dynasty.* New York: Knopf, 1978.

Wright, David. *Translating Science: The Transmission of Western Chemistry into Late Imperial China, 1840–1900.* Leiden: Brill, 2000.

———. "The Translation of Modern Western Science in Nineteenth-Century China, 1840–1895." *Isis* 89.4 (1998): 653–673.

Wu, Hong-zhou, Panji Cheng, and Zhaoqin Fan. *Fundamentals of Traditional Chinese Medicine.* Hackensack, NJ: World Century Publishing, 2013.

Wu, Lien-teh and Sung Chih-ai. "Huo-luan: A Study of This Syndrome and Its Relations to Cholera Asiatica." *Reports of the National Quarantine Service* Series 4 (1933): 1–16.

Wu, Yi-li. "Bodily Knowledge and Western Learning in Late Imperial China: The Case of Wang Shixiong (1808–68)." In Howard Chiang, editor, *Historical Epistemology and the Making of Modern Chinese Medicine,* 80–112. Manchester, UK: Manchester University Press, 2015.

———. *Reproducing Women: Medicine, Metaphor, and Childbirth in Late Imperial China.* Berkeley: University of California Press, 2010.

Xie Guan. *Zhong guo yi xue yuan liu lun* [On the origins of Chinese medicine]. Shanghai: Shanghai Zhongyi shuju, 1935.

———. *Zhong yi da ci dian* [Great Dictionary of Chinese Medicine]. 1921. Beijing: Shangwu yinshuguan guoji youxian gongsi, 2003.

Yan Jianhua. "Zhong yi you shi bing zhong zhuan jia diao cha ji qi li lun tan yuan [A survey of experts concerning the types of diseases that Chinese medicine is especially good for]." *Jiangsu Zhongyi* 22.9 (2001): 1–4.

Yan Jinghui, "Ying you er nao xing jiao qi bing CT zhen duan fen xi ji jian bie zhen duan [Differential diagnosis and CT diagnostic analysis of neurological beriberi in infants]," *Dangdai yixue* 19.4.303 (February 2013): 113–114.

Yang, Bin. "The Zhang on Chinese Southern Frontiers: Disease Constructions, Environmental Changes, and Imperial Colonization." *Bulletin of the History of Medicine* 84.2 (2010): 163–192.

Yamada Keiji. *The Origins of Acupuncture, Moxibustion, and Decoction.* Kyoto: International Research Center for Japanese Studies, 1998.

Yamashita Seizō. *Kakke no rekishi: bitamin hakken izen.* [History of foot qi: before the discovery of vitamins]. Tokyo: Tokyo daigaku shuppansha, 1983.

Yang, Rae. *Spider Eaters: A Memoir.* Berkeley: University of California Press, 2013.

Yu Tuan. *Xin bian yi xue zheng chuan* [Newly compiled Orthodox transmission of medical knowledge]. 1515. In the *Xu xiu si ku quan shu*, v. 1019, 241–546. Shanghai: Shanghai guji chubanshe, 1995.

Yuan Bing. *"Song dai fang ji xue cheng jiu yu te dian yan jiu (960–1279 AD)* [Research on the achievements and special characteristics of pharmacology in the Song dynasty (960–1279 AD)]." Master's thesis. Beijing: Zhongyi yanjiu yuan, 2002.

Yule, Henry. *Hobson-Jobson: A Glossary of Colloquial Anglo-Indian Words and Phrases, and of Kindred Terms, Etymological, Historical, Geographical and Discursive.* New edition edited by William Crooke. London: J. Murray, 1903.

"Yun fu you jiao qi qian wan bie luan yong yao [Pregnant foot qi sufferers must not recklessly use medicine]." 39 Yu'er Pindao. Retrieved on March 23, 2017, from http://baby.39.net/a/140927/4481265.html.

Zeng Chaoran. *Jiao qi chu yan* [Superficial remarks on foot *qi*]. Guangzhou: Guangzhou ju zhen tang, 1887.

Zeng Shirong. *Huo you kou yi* [Oral comments on saving children's lives]. 1332. Beijing: Zhongyi guji chubanshe, 1985.

Zhan, Mei. *Other-Worldly: Making Chinese Medicine through Transnational Frames.* Durham, NC: Duke University Press, 2009.

Zhang Canjia. *Zhong yi gu ji wen xian xue* [The study of ancient books and documents in Chinese medicine]. Beijing: Renmin weisheng chubanshe, 1998.

Zhang Congzheng. *Ru men shi qin* [A scholar's service to his parents]. 1224–1231. In *Zi he yi ji*, edited by Deng Tietao et al. Beijing: Ren min wei sheng chu ban she, 1994.

Zhang Daqing. "Gao si lan: yi xue ming ci fan yi biao zhun hua de tui dong zhe [Cousland: promoter of standardized translations for medical terms]." *Zhongguo keji shiliao* 22.4 (2001): 224–230.

————. *Zhong guo jin dai ji bing she hui shi (1912–1937)* [A social history of diseases in modern China]. Jinan: Shandong jiaoyu chubanshe, 2006.

Zhang Gang. *Zhong yi bai bing ming yuan kao* [Study of the origins of disease names in Chinese medicine]. Beijing: Renmin weisheng chubanshe, 1997.

Zhang Hefen. *Jiao qi zheng ji yao* [Summary of the symptoms of foot *qi*]. 1909. First edition, held in the library of the Zhongyi kexue yuan in Beijing.

Zhang Jiebin. *Jing Yue quan shu* [Collected works of Jing Yue (aka Zhang Jiebin)]. Beijing: Renmin weisheng chubanshe, 2007.

Zhang Shiche. *Ji jiu liang fang* [Excellent formulas for rescuing people in emergency situations]. 1550. In *Zhongguo yixue da cheng san bian*, vol. 4. Edited by Qiu Peiran. Changsha: Yue lu shu she, 1994.

Zhang Shuhua, Wang Zengzhen, and Liu Guoxia. "Zhong yao si fen san zhi liao jiao qi 47 li [47 cases of foot qi treated with four powdered Chinese drugs]." *Zhongguo min jian liaofa* (China's Naturopathy) 20.11 (November 2012): 16–17.

Zhang Zaitong and Xian Rijin, eds. *Min guo yi yao wei sheng fa gui xuan bian (1912–1948)* [Selected laws and regulations from the Republic of China regarding medicine and public health]. Ji'nan: Shandong daxue chubanshe, 1990.

Zhong yi yao xue ming ci shen ding wei yuan hui [Committee to examine and approve Chinese medicine and pharmacy terminology]. *Zhong yi yao xue ming ci* [Chinese terms in Traditional Chinese Medicine and pharmacy]. Beijing: Kexue chubanshe, 2004.

Zhu Su. *Pu ji fang* [Universal aid formulary]. 1406. Beijing: Renmin weisheng chubanshe, 1983.

Index

9 781503 603448